Somewhere In A Rainbow

Living in a world with a mental or substance problem is like living in a world of unconscious and conscious paranoia and loneliness.

I0105069

RASHEEDAH SHARIF

"What would you do if you were high in the mountains, in a tiny room with no windows or doors?"

Dedicated to my eight children.

Thank you

Thank you to my daughter, Chinue Sharif, for taking the time, energy and love to edit my story.

I imagine this was a challenging experience due to me being her mother.

She assured me that it would not be a problem.

My faith and blessings went with her spirit as she took the journey into my past.

Thank you, my Chi.

Thank you to my six children: Shakira, Maryam, Ab, Yaya, Imani and Chinue.

Your contributions to the about the author, your mother, is a book within itself.

I am honored to be your mother. You have been with me throughout your entire lives.

Your unconditional love for me was the energy that gave me the will to want to live.

You are the greatest blessings I have received in my life.

May the angels continue to lift your wings as you continue to soar toward heaven.

Ma'Me

TABLE OF CONTENTS

PART ONE

INTRODUCTION

"It's lonely and frightening inside. I'm embarrassed and ashamed to tell anyone how I am really feeling. I don't want the stigma of being weak or always complaining.

Besides, people come to me for help. What would it look like if I ran to someone for help?

I can't put my stuff out like that!"

Living in a world with a mental or substance problem is like living in a world of unconscious and conscious paranoia and loneliness.

We know something is wrong, but we don't know how to think about it because our emotions are directly attached and precedes rational thoughts.

We are stigmatized for being different by family, friends, religious congregations and educational family. Our circle of people who are supposed to keep us safe and help us to evolve into positive adults are triggers to our emotions. We hide our depression, anxiety, aggression and other mental disturbances.

In addition, we are often clueless as to *why* we feel so disconnected from our self and others.

In an attempt to *not* think about the *something* or societal stigmas, we numb our emotions with a variety of outlets that creates a false sense of happiness and success.

Substances, sex, violence, workaholism, an unhealthy overindulgence in religion and other outlets are choices that covers the real issue.

Besides, who doesn't enjoy sex and the belief that religion equals faith, right?

Overindulgence in a behavior in order to create a temporary feeling of euphoria, perpetuates denial and avoidance.

Twenty-one days of a particular behavior creates a habit.

What role do societal stigmas play in preventing a person from getting help with a mental or substance problem?

This is a true account of my story.

Rose

There is a history of sexual abuse, domestic violence, drug and alcohol abuse throughout the years of preadolescence into adulthood. The behavior went unnoticed and untreated.

At age sixteen Rose left home to live with her eighteen-year aged boyfriend.

She became a teen mother at age sixteen, and by her twentieth birthday, she had given birth to four babies.

By age sixty-five, Rose was stressed, depressed and her blood pressure was not stabilized.

Her doctor told her to go on an extended vacation for at least a year. Rose decided to retire.

Within a couple of months, she began to feel better. She began to do simple things to make her happy.

Rose retired in March of 2018. In July of 2018, she became the sole caregiver of her mother.

The circumstances surrounding the need for Rose to care for her mother sent her into a state of depression and feelings of hopelessness.

Past abuses materialized in her thoughts. Without warning, she began to have nightmares about sexual and domestic violence.

She discovered that her mother's and her life paralleled the history of domestic violence and sexual abuse.

Hearing repeated stories of the graphic abuse her mother survived, Rose fell into a state of depression. Her nightmares increased and insomnia was the norm.

Triggers are exploding and her mental and physical stability is challenged.

Rose is in a place of darkness and feels hopeless.

Here are the reasons I am motivated to share my story.

- *To dispel the myth that therapy is for 'crazy' people.*

- *To help alleviate the stigmas and low self-worth generated by society.*

- *To learn what 'triggers' are through self-awareness.*

- *To dismiss the belief that your stuff is so unique that no one else is experiencing it or will understand what you are going through.*

- *To help individuals to simply relax and embrace the idea that there is someone capable of helping them through a crisis.*

- *To communicate to all people that they are worthy of getting better, capable of feeling better and have the ability to do better.*

- *To encourage people to take that extra step in finding a qualified professional.*

It took Rose sixty-five years to realize that getting professional help was okay.

SESSION #1

———— ∿ ————

Strong oak tree up high

Never bends so majestic

Oak tree breaks and dies.

Therapist

Tell me, why you are here, Rose?

Rose

I thought I was able to handle my feelings on my own, but every day I wake up I feel hopeless. Here we are in Spring 2020 and all that I can think about is not catching the Corona virus aka COVID-19. This virus seems to have appeared out of nowhere! It's so new that the scientists and medical professionals are stumbling in the dark trying to find out how to control it.

I am the caregiver of my mother; she's ninety-two. It frightens me that she is in the age and health category of being at risk for having grave consequences if she catches it. I'm in the age category as well. She has asthma, recovered from breast cancer surgery in 2008, hypertension, had the flu and pneumonia. She is very vulnerable. It worries me!

I am also frightened for my children and their families. It concerns me that they feel invincible to this virus and are not taking it seriously.

The CDC has announced that it does not affect the young as much as the elderly and folks with health issues. They are saying if you are 65 and over, and have health issues such as diabetes, heart problems, high blood pressure and respiratory issues, that you stand a higher risk of catching the virus. Hell, that's over half of the population! There is a tremendous amount of mental pressure on me to keep myself safe; almost to the point of becoming paranoid. I need to be healthy to care for my mother and I don't want my children to be without their mother if I get it and die. I have two sons I have not seen since 2005 and one son that is in prison. I have to push back my emotions when the thought of not knowing about their circumstances or where they are invades my mind and creates fear.

The CDC has issued guidelines for the entire nation. Those guidelines include distancing yourself from loved ones and all people, wear a mask when in public, use hand sanitizer when out and about and wash your hands as often as you can. They call it *social distancing*. That term evokes loneliness. Who wants to be constantly reminded that they cannot have any social interaction? I wonder why they didn't say, *physical distancing*? Physical distancing has more of a doable ring to it and sounds less mentally depressing to the spirit. They have also mandated for people to shelter in place. We are not allowed to go anywhere unless it is essential. That includes no visits to our family member's homes. Whoever you are with indoors, you will have to be in there with them for a period of two weeks. Most folks are calling it, *lock-down*. The two weeks are supposed to determine if you display any symptoms.

This two-week period has transformed into more than fourteen days of sheltering in place, aka lock-down. Again, the term lock-down is so damn negative.

All businesses have been closed, the beaches are closed and the only businesses that remain open are pharmacies, grocery stores, gas stations and banks. The medical institutions are overwhelmed, nurses, doctors, police officers, firefighters and first responders are contracting the virus. Some live but many are dying. We do not have any leadership at the national level. States are doing different things and there is no unity among the United States!

This entire situation is depressing. What's so interesting is, it's not only COVID-19 that's got me stressed. COVID-19 is the straw that broke the camel's back.

I need to be here.

Therapist

You are caring for yourself and your mother enough to come. That's great!

Let's talk about whatever you want to talk about. Let's eliminate the traditional beginning, middle or end. You have already begun. Wherever you are with your story is your beginning.

I would like you to talk about the things you feel have impacted you the most.

Rose

Ok. I can do that. But let me hear who you are? It feels uncomfortable spilling my life out to a stranger. I need to feel comfortable with telling you about the real issues I am having without holding back.

Therapist

Fair enough! First of all, your journey towards healing began before you came to see me. Let me be the first to congratulate you on making the decision.

Just so you know, all of the decisions you have made in your life have been just that, decisions. We will not label them right or wrong.

However, for every so-called wrong decision, there has been a life lesson attached to it. There have been times you get it and feel good about the decision and there have been times you didn't get it and felt uncomfortable. The great thing about life is that we get another opportunity to do it over again; providing we take advantage of the opportunity. You'll discover that for every decision we make in life, it will lead you to another and then another. With each decision we make, we grow a little more. In some cases, we keep repeating the same lessons.

Welcome to moving forward with your life and discovering new ways to make different types of decisions.

Talking with someone else up front and close means they will see me.

Rose

I want to be perfectly honest with you. A lot of decisions I have made in the past have been good and some not so good. I feel bad that I have allowed myself to not be a priority in certain ways. Sometimes I wish I had more of a 'I don't care' attitude. Maybe I wouldn't feel so hopeless. I feel hopeless. There, I said it! I feel hopeless!

Therapist

What does that feel like?

Rose

I thought I had everything under control.

Therapist

Control?

Rose

Yes. I mean my past. I have been having nightmares. I am experiencing a lot of anxiety and fear. I panic about things I would not normally panic about and I am always tired. Not tired from doing things, just plain tired. I'm about to twist my hair out of my head and it is becoming increasingly hard for me to relax during certain situations.

I feel hopeless about my life and I am not happy. Meditation isn't working. Well, it works for the moment, but then my mind goes back to my current situation. I am unable to cut through those thoughts of a future that is worse than today. I can't even cry. My thoughts and current situation are defeating me. I am here because I do not want to resort to my old habit of self-medicating. I have a history of self-medicating. You know, drugs! Self-medicating sounds better, but the bottom line, it's substance abuse.

The way I feel is similar to how I felt in the past just before I began self-medicating. Only now, I am aware of it and it makes me feel worse.

I want to live, travel, have fun and be carefree to do what I want. I want to put me as a priority.

I can't see it or feel it. I feel trapped in a circle of sadness and hopelessness.

My dreams aren't in color, anymore. I wake up feeling tired, wishing I could go back and get some real quality sleep. It's not happening for me.

I can't feel the rainbow.

LIFE PATH

———— ～～～ ————

Dawn born with red ray

Riant eyes sparkled at night

Death became her friend

Rose

- Rose was born on a Wednesday, September 22 to the parents of Helen and Grover Smith.

- When she was born her older sister was six years, one brother of three years and another of two years.

- She states that her first memory was at age three of twin girls dressed in brightly colored sun rompers. This stands out in her mind due to her imagining they were her children to care for.

- Rose states that her mother shared with her that she was grown before her time. It amazed her that a child who could not walk tried to teach and tell her what to say. Her mother shared to Rose that before she would go to sleep at night, her mother would have to say, "good night suga." Her first babysitter was an elderly woman with snow white hair. Rose says that she and the woman had conversations as if they were best friends. Rose recalls large tubs of green ferns surrounding the perimeter of the babysitter's porch. Rose remembers that she would always fall off the porch and into the lush green ferns.

- Rose states that she was sexually abused at age five. The abuse happened when her mother left her father. She and her mother took temporary residence with a woman friend of her mother's. The friend had three children. One daughter about 12 to 13 years and two brothers around 9 and 10 years. Rose states that they sexually abused her for the duration of the time they stayed there. She does not recall how long they were there. Rose did not mention to her mother or siblings about what happened. No one found out.

- At age five, Rose's parents separated permanently, and they later divorced. She blamed herself for the separation. Rose remembers that she cried to her father about what her mother and grandmother discussed. They said, they would have him locked up if he put his hands on her mother again.

- Age five, she and family relocated to Jasper, FL from Jacksonville, FL to live with grandparents. Rose's parents divorced. Rose's father went to prison for lack of child support.

- Age six, Rose's father sent her a doll dressed in a long lace white wedding dress. She listened as her grandmother and mother made the decision for her, to send the doll back to her father. Rose states that she really wanted the doll and that she cried all night in her bed.

- Rose began school at age six. She states that the school was all black due to racial segregation. Her first experience was black teachers' cruel treatment towards children who had dark skin and girls with short hair. The teachers grouped those children together and sat them in the back of the class. Rose stated that the teachers made a daily *sport* of keeping her and other dark-skinned students after school to beat them on their hands with a thick strip of tire. She never told her mother or grandmother. She recalls open segregation in the town. Black people could not sit in the same movie section, eat at the same restaurants or drink from the same water fountains. While in a store, white people would follow you around as if you were a thief, Rose states. She recalls going on errands with her sister in a part of town where white people lived. The white people would sic their dogs on her and her sister. She recalls learning the pledge of allegiance and Tom, Dick and Jane stories in her first-grade books.

- Age six, her mother gave birth to a boy. This was six years and one day after her birthday. She remembers being happy and wanting to take care of the baby.

- Age seven, Rose created dolls to play with made from soda bottles for the body, corn silk for the hair and quilt swatches for the clothes. She states the dolls were her babies.

- Age eight, her older sister relocated to Newark, NJ to live with their aunt and first cousin, Cher. The first cousin was a girl, age ten. The intention was for her sister to get a better education in the North. Rose felt alone and that her first cousin was replacing her. She states that her brothers did not pay her any attention because they had each other. She adds, her baby brother was off limits to her. It was her older brother's responsibility to look after him, she was too young.

- Age eight, Rose lost her best friend, Wilbur. He was her chocolate, stuffed teddy bear. After losing him she formed a bond with a Chinaberry tree.

- Age ten, Rose, her three brothers ages four, twelve and thirteen, and mother relocated to Newark, NJ. The family took the Greyhound Bus. She recalls getting sick from eating hot-dogs and throwing up during the trip.

- Age ten, upon arriving to NJ, Rose recalls being separated from her mother. She lived with an adult cousin, husband and their three-year-old daughter. They lived on Fairmont Avenue, Newark, NJ. She states she did not have prior knowledge of the living situation. Rose experienced nightmares and sleep walking almost every night. Her reoccurring dream was her becoming a spider. Her adult cousin would come into the room during the nightmares and find her climbing on the wall. Other times, she would get out of bed and go and have conversations with her cousins only to be awaken by them and confused.

- Age ten, Rose was bussed to Burnet Street School. She recalls being bullied on and off the bus. Her milk money was taken from her each day. Rose did not tell anyone. She states that the school had white teachers, and this was her first experience interacting with white people. Rose heard curse words for the first time. She could not identify with the children and did not make any friends.

- Age ten, Rose learned nasty-worded steps and played french and double dutch jump rope when outside. The only way she could fit in was to say the nasty step words and do the steps. Rose states she became good at jumping rope.

- Age eleven, Rose's mother found an apartment for the family; sister and three brothers. Although she was happy with the fact that her family was reuniting, she says she always felt alone, scared and lost.

- Age eleven, Rose was greeted by a boy three years older and a girl from her class who was a year older. This happened after school in a confined hallway. They jumped her, with him delivering the most damage. She recalls getting punched in the nose so hard until she cried like a baby. She ran home crying. Her brother, who was two years older than her, went to the school but the school doors were locked. That was the end of that.

- Age twelve, Rose states that she was sexually molested by an adult family member. She did not tell anyone because she thought she did something wrong and did not want to cause a problem.

- Age twelve, Rose began to take pills and drink alcohol while in school. Bacardi and Coke and Colt 45 were the drinks of choice. The pills made her nod. Rose would cut classes and play "hooky" from school. She and a group of girls would hang out in the basement of one of the students or go on the rooftop of the projects on Mercer Street. She'd get so drunk that it caused her to throw up. She'd tell herself that she wouldn't drink again but always did. She states that pills and alcohol made her laugh and have fun with her friends. This was the only time she was happy. She attended West Kinney Junior High School.

- Age thirteen, Rose witnessed the riots in Newark, NJ. At first, people were protesting the brutality. Violence erupted and rioting behavior dominated the streets. She watched as her neighborhood was burned down. She recalls army tanks, machine guns, fires, looting and a fearful mother. She observed police and other authority figures beat people to the ground. She recalls hearing gunshots throughout the day and night. She watched looters run up and down the street with arms filled with merchandise taken from stores. Rose states she was not afraid and did not understand why she and her brothers couldn't go out and loot the stores. Rose states that the message for why the protest began was lost and people were not heard. A cab driver had gotten killed by a cop and that was the last straw for the community. Nothing was made of the fact that the cab driver lost his life. She states, it was as if the reason for the protest had been burned in the fires.

- Age fourteen, Rose barley goes to school. She signs in and leaves the premises. She associates with a group of friends, including her first cousin Cher, who goes to the home of a lady who is in her early twenties. They drink, play music, dance and sing. There are no sexual acts involved with the group, who later allows three boys to attend the parties. She attended West Side High School.

- Age fifteen, Rose is rescued by a boy who spots her while on the corner of her high school hang out. She is throwing up and alone. The boy becomes her good friend. She feels safe and cared for when in his presence. She states this is the first time she felt someone looking at her and caring for her with no strings attached. The friendship dissolves when summer arrived. She has periodic dreams about the boy who rescued her off the corner. Rose believes he is her soul mate.

- Age fifteen, Rose met a boy who was two years older. She says he was known as a bad boy. He became her boyfriend. He bossed her around and told her everything to do. This is what she thought love was all about. He'd talk her into missing school and take her to his residence and discuss the type of girl he wanted to be with. He'd also tell her about his experience when he went to the Youth House. It was a juvenile detention facility for children who had gotten into trouble by breaking the law.

- Age fifteen, her boyfriend began to slap her in the face. He told her he did it because he loved her. Her girlfriends shared this belief. She thought he loved her.

- Age fifteen, Rose was introduced to Islam by her boyfriend. In order to remain his girlfriend, she had to become a Muslim and become a member of the Nation of Islam. She had to learn the Actual Facts and Student Enrollment before becoming a registered member. Her boyfriend did not allow her to go to the Mosque and formally register. He began to control everything she did; the food she ate, the clothes she wore, who she could hang out with, when and where she went and what she should say to her mother. She felt sad and unhappy all the time. She states that she did not know how to talk to anyone about what she felt. He told her to stop smiling because there was nothing to smile about, according to the Honorable Elijah Muhammad. She thought her boyfriend loved her because he hit her and was telling her everything to do.

- Age fifteen, Rose's mother forbade her to see him and she had to stop wearing long skirts and scarves, as required by the Nation of Islam. She and her mother grew further apart. She felt unhappy, alone, trapped and did not know what to do. She did not have anyone to confide in or talk to. Rose ran away from home to live with her boyfriend, at his request.

- In about two weeks, her mother came and got her from where she was staying. She states that her mother did not discuss or ask why she had left home.

- Age fifteen, Rose gets a Morse sewing machine from Sun Sewing Company on Bradford Street, Newark, NJ. She states, the sewing machine went wherever she went. She parted with the machine in 2005.

- Age fifteen, she and boyfriend made a plan for her to get pregnant. She thought that this would be her way to leave home. She states that her mother would disown her if she got pregnant. Rose got pregnant. Her mother gave in to the fact that

Rose was going to do what she wanted and agreed to let her move in with her boyfriend. Her mother would be remarrying and relocating to Rochester, NJ during the same time.

- Age sixteen, Rose leaves home. She and boyfriend get an apartment together on Beacon Street, Newark, NJ. It was a cold-water flat. Two tiny rooms, bathroom, small kitchen and a large hot water tank that sat in the kitchen. The hot water tank also served as a heater for the winter. The apartment was located in the back of some buildings that sat on the front side of the street.

- Age sixteen, the physical abuse escalates. Rose states that boyfriend is now punching her and promises to really "fuck" her up when she has the baby. Nevertheless, he still slapped her around during her pregnancy.

- Age sixteen, Rose delivers a baby girl. Baby girl was born on Good Friday. Her mother came to visit and was present for the birth. For the first time in her life she feels a rush of happiness and love that she has never felt before. Domestic violence escalates. She does not tell anyone.

- Age sixteen, within six weeks of birth, she gets pregnant with a second child. The sex was not welcomed. The verbal and physical abuse is unbearable.

- Age seventeen, Rose delivers her second child, alone in the hospital. She has a 5lb son.

- Age seventeen, Rose states that the abuse is extreme, and she never gets enough to eat. She feeds the babies mashed navy beans and canned milk. She borrows canned milk from her sister. There is no one to talk to. Her boyfriend threatened to beat anyone up if she told what goes on inside the house.

- Age eighteen, she contacts her mother and makes a plan to leave her boyfriend and go to Rochester, NY to stay with her mother, youngest brother and mother's husband. She arrives and stays for two months. She does not recall talking to her mother about the abuse she endured.

- Age eighteen, she gets financial assistance from the county and gets her own apartment. Her children are ages one and two. Rose becomes active within the Nation of Islam.

- Age eighteen, she gets lonely and gets back with her boyfriend. He comes to Rochester. She felt sorry for herself and her children. She wanted her children to have their father. He convinces her this is the right thing to do. They get back together in less than six months after her leaving. Within a few weeks the physical violence resumed.

- Age eighteen, she and her boyfriend legally marry. Her involvement with the Nation of Islam required a marriage certificate. She did not want to get married. The marriage was performed by the Justice of the Peace. She became pregnant with a third child.

- Age eighteen and pregnant, the first doctor's appointment reveals a sexually transmitted disease. The abuse escalated. He openly expressed anger in words and physical abuse because she left him.

- Age nineteen, Rose birthed a boy. Her mother worked at the same hospital where she gave birth. She does not recall many details about the pregnancy or delivery.

- Age nineteen, Rose states all she wanted to do was sleep. Rose recalls struggling to care for her three children and enduring domestic violence from her husband. She did not confide in anyone and no longer attended the Mosque. Within two months, she is pregnant with a fourth child.

- Age nineteen, she asks her mother for help. She and her mother make a plan for her to leave and relocate to Jasper, FL. The plan was for her to stay with her grandmother until she could get on her feet. She left Rochester with her three children, ages three, two and under a year, along with her Morse sewing machine.

- Age nineteen, in her seventh month of pregnancy she moved into a low-income community. After living there for a month, Rose states she became afraid and lonely. She contacts her husband. He convinces her to take him back so that he could help with the children. She takes him back.

- Age twenty and under extreme duress, she delivers her fourth child, a girl, in Jasper, FL. She states that her wrist and ankles were strapped down to the delivery bed.

- Age twenty, Rose and her husband make arrangements to return to Newark, NJ.

- Age twenty, she and her four children, ages three months to four years, live with multiple families. The family living in the projects on Mercy Street was where she and her family lived until they moved on Goldsmith Avenue in Newark, NJ. Her husband lived elsewhere. She states that three of her children slept in one bunk bed and she and her three-month old baby slept in another bunk bed. She states in order to stay out of the family's way, they remained in the room most of the time. Rose recalls falling asleep while cooking and the entire apartment filling with smoke; there were no smoke detectors. She recalls always being hungry and that any food she had, she gave it to her children. She did not have an income at that time, she states. She was totally dependent on her abusive husband.

- Age twenty, Rose moves in with a Muslim family on

Goldsmith Avenue in Newark, NJ. She states that for the first time she feels safe.

- Age twenty, Rose gets an apartment in the Muslim family's home that is located on the first floor. Rose met a family who lived next door. She states that they were kind and loving beyond words to her children and her. She states she and her children had never been embraced with such warmth and non-judgmental love. Rose has made up her mind to not allow her husband to return under any circumstances.

- Age twenty, Rose feels certain that her abuser will not beat her while she is in the home of Muslims. She states that he comes around at night and knocks on the door and window seeking to get in.

- Age twenty-one, her husband forces his way into her apartment and forces himself on her sexually.

- Age twenty-one, Rose goes to Beth Israel Hospital to have an abortion. Rose states that one of the daughters who lived next door volunteered at the same hospital. She holds Rose by the hand and guides her through the emotional impact of having an abortion. Afterwards, she and the neighbor become close friends. The neighbor helps her with her four children.

- Age twenty-one, Rose's two oldest children are taken from a daycare center by her abuser. She states, this was his attempt to make her take him back. He'd call on the phone and the children would be crying for her. She became detective and told the police the story. The police and Rose went to the apartment where he was holding the children. She took her children home.

- Age twenty-one, her abuser abducted her. He was waiting in the back seat of a taxicab as she was making her way to the hospital to see her oldest son. Her son had a hernia and was recovering after surgery, Rose states. The cab driver was a high school friend. He was giving her a ride, off the records. When she entered the cab, a pair of hands from the front seat grabbed her neck and began to choke and shake her. Her friend didn't do anything. He followed the instructions of the abuser. Rose states, she must have passed out. She recalls being on a roof top of a building without any clothes on. He was threatening to push her off if she didn't take him back. Rose does not recall how it ended.

- Age twenty-one, Rose states that she seeks help. She contacts an associate and puts in place a way for him to get shot and killed. The contract fell through.

- Age twenty-one, Rose starts going to the Mosque. This is where she met S. Rose states that she was an angel who took her under her wing as a big sister. S had two children and was looking for a sitter for her four-year old son. Rose decided to become a sitter. Rose became a sitter and made clothes for children and women to supplement her welfare check.

- Age twenty-one, Rose's income is not able to pay the rent and care for her children. She has to move.

- Age twenty-one, Rose is invited to live with S. S and her two children, a daughter aged ten and son aged four, lived in the Weequahic Towers in Newark, NJ.

- Age twenty-one, Rose met a Muslim by the name of Rasheed. He was the brother of the Muslim family on Goldsmith Avenue. He would visit the family from time to time. She desperately wanted to be with him all the time. She was attracted to his courage and strength. He did not allow Rose to get close. He treated her like a sister.

- Age twenty-one, she did not hear or see him again. She changed her name to match his name.

- Age twenty-one, Rose got a divorce from her abuser. The county paid for the divorce.

- Age twenty-one, she met the love of her life. He was a real man, she states. She says he provided for and protected her children and her without hesitation.

- They became great companions. They got their own apartment in the Weequahic Towers. Rose became pregnant and had a fifth child at age twenty-two.

- Age twenty-two, he and Rose were married.

- Age twenty-two, Rose is pregnant with a sixth child.

- Age twenty-two, her husband went to Danbury Correctional Facility for three years.

- Age twenty-three, Rose gave birth to a premature baby girl.

- Age twenty-three, Rose relocated to Albany, GA to live with in-laws until she could regain her emotions. Conditions became unfavorable when she was laid off from her job.

- Age twenty-four, she relocated back to Newark, NJ after living in Albany, GA for less than a year. She eventually moves into a three-family home located in Irvington, NJ.

- Age twenty-five, her husband went back prison. He was convicted of a bank robbery and sentenced to sixty years.

- Age twenty-five, Rose got her first job at a fast food restaurant in Irvington, NJ.

- Age twenty-six, Rose was evicted from her apartment in Irvington.

- Age twenty-five, Rose and her six children, ages three through ten, moved to a basement apartment on Shanley Avenue in Newark, NJ. She states they slept on two mattresses on a cold and damp basement floor for six months.

- Age twenty-five, Rose made the decision to start college. She enrolled in a Women's Program at Bloomfield College. She attended classes in the evening.

- Age twenty-six, Rose and children moved to South Munn Avenue in East Orange, NJ.

- Age twenty-seven, Rose began to use cocaine, marijuana and drank Guinness Stout.

- Age twenty-nine, Rose is physically assaulted and nearly raped while on her way home from an evening class at Bloomfield College. She states therapy did not help. She withdrew from night classes for a semester and began day classes. Her use of substances increased.

- Age thirty, Rose became a member of the Ausar Auset Society, an Ancient Kemetic Meditation organization that was based in Brooklyn, NY. She learned the ancient art of meditation.

- Age thirty-one, Rose earned a Bachelor's degree from Bloomfield College. Her mother, children, sister and close friends attended her graduation.

- Age thirty-one, Rose began to teach full-time at New-Ark School in Newark, NJ. She states that she was exposed to a world of culture which enabled her to express creativity.

- Age thirty-one, Rose was formally taught color therapy. Her teacher was an elder stranger she met while at Gino's Restaurant in downtown Newark, NJ. After nine months of intense lessons, he dropped out of her life.

- Age thirty-one, Rose met another man she believed to have loved. Rose conceived her seventh pregnancy.

- Age thirty-two, Rose taught in the public-school system. Rose was involved in community affairs and served as a county community member. Rose created a drama ensemble with the neighborhood children. The children performed plays at various locations.

- Age thirty-two, Rose's relationship with the new man ended. The breakup occurred during her third trimester of pregnancy. Rose gave birth to a baby boy and went back to work in the school system when the baby was a few weeks.

- Ages thirty-two to thirty-seven, Rose cared for her children and continued to work as a teacher in the public-school system.

- Age thirty-seven Rose met another man she believed to love and conceived child number eight.

- Age thirty-eight, Rose gave birth to a baby girl. Rose went back to work in the school system when the baby was two weeks.

- Age thirty-nine, Rose met Mr. Robert Richie. He taught her how to sculpt trees from wire. Rose recalls him coming into her life and suddenly disappearing after teaching her the art.

- Age forty, Rose's grandmother who lived in Jasper, Florida became ill. Rose was asked to relocate so that someone could live in her grandmother's home. Rose and her three youngest children relocated to Jasper, Florida.

- Age forty, Rose began work as a high school teacher at a juvenile detention center in Hamilton County. She taught history, drama and English. She created and facilitated a student written publication entitled, Dare to Rise.

- Age forty-two, Rose relocated to Tallahassee, FL after feeling too closed in from living in a small town. She recalls needing more opportunities for her children and herself.

- Age forty-two, Rose counseled women in relapse prevention at a women's correctional facility in Jefferson County, Florida.

- Age fifty, Rose undergoes chemotherapy. She does not remember a lot about the experience. She states that she went on her first cruise and ignored the treatment while away. Her oldest son came for an extended visit during that time. He brought two of his children and partner with him. Rose's second son performed nurse duties. She states she was afraid, and he reassured her all would be well. Rose's eldest daughter was her right hand and never left her side. Rose states, the two of them still joke about the hard microwave toast she made after finding out Rose was hungry.

- Age fifty-one, Rose relocates to Tampa, Florida with her youngest child. Rose states she wanted a fresh start and to live in a location that was not reliant on seasonal activities. Ybor City in Tampa convinced her that she was making a good choice.

- Ages fifty-one through sixty, Rose volunteers for a domestic violence shelter, The Spring of Tampa Bay. She attends classes and gets certified as a domestic violence advocate.

- Age fifty-six, Rose purchases a townhome in Tampa, FL.

- Age fifty-seven, Rose writes and publishes her first book in a memoir entitled, *Don't Come Down from the Chinaberry Tree*.

- Age fifty-seven, while working at an Exceptional Student Center for students with emotional behavioral disturbances, Rose starts a Master's program at Grand Canyon University.

- Age fifty-seven, Rose starts and completes her internship at the Phoenix House Addiction Treatment Center.

- Age fifty-nine, Rose earns a master's degree in Addictions Counseling from Grand Canyon University.

- Age fifty-nine, Rose starts work at DAACO Behavioral Health Residential Treatment for Women.

- Age sixty-one, Rose gets a white Maltese puppy. She names him Winter.

- Age sixty-one, Rose downsizes her life and moves from her home. She and her puppy relocate to a studio apartment in Clearwater Beach, Florida.

- Age sixty-one, Rose gets a job at Paul B. Stevens Center. The school cares for students with profound physical disabilities.

- Age sixty-one, Rose makes the decision to find Winter a new home. She states that she is still working, overwhelmed and could not care for him properly.

- Age sixty-three, Rose's doctor recommends an early retirement due to stress and anxiety from the job. Rose's doctor recommended a vacation frame of mind for at least one year.

- Age sixty-three, Rose becomes the care giver of her 90-year-old mother. She travels to Rochester, NY to get her. They reside in the studio apartment. Within two months Rose moves to an upstairs apartment.

- Age sixty-four, Rose and mother relocate to a two-bedroom condominium in Deerfield Beach, Florida.

- Age sixty-five, life in quarantine with her elderly mother, as they adapt to living with the reality of COVID-19.

Session #2

Rose

I am unable to sleep. I have nightmares about the past abuse in my life. I sometimes wake to someone pushing me off the roof of the projects.

Therapist

The projects roof?

Rose

Yes, once that asshole took me up to the roof and made me take my clothes off. He then threatened to push me off.

Therapist

Rose, tell me how you are feeling?

Rose

I am feeling like I took a crazy pill.

I am about to twist my hair out. It's hard for me to stop, so I think I'll just cut it all off. I have to put a hat on my head to help me to stop.

I wake up in the morning, still tired. During the day all I want to do is sleep.

I sometimes feel guilty that I want to be by myself and not be bothered.

My mother and I live together, you know. I want to be alone but I know she needs me. I do not see a way for me to get better or to feel better.

I feel like there is no light at the end of the tunnel. It's a feeling of hopelessness; like a double-edged sword. Currently, I am dealing with the fact that my mother has been traumatized all her life and that her third husband nearly killed her. That picture floats around in my head. Her trauma experience and mine are sort of merging together. Her stuff has triggered my stuff to the surface. She talks about it every day! The conversations are our sunrise and my sunset. I try to redirect the conversation to something else, but that lasts for only a split second. Then, out of her head to her mouth comes the mention of death, beatings and abuse all over again. I feel so sorry for her. I lie in bed thinking about that shit. It floods my thoughts whether I'm awake or asleep. I am restless, tired, anxious and my stomach is in knots.

I feel sad all day! I worry about my mother. I know that she needs to get it out. Hell, you're talking about ninety years of abuse! Her health is declining and her cognition is not the same.

I try to remember what it was like when I was a child but there isn't any memory. I sometimes, well, often times do not have energy to do anything but watch TV. I feel like taking a drink of wine to help me to sleep or to take the edge off my sadness. God knows I don't want to do that. I don't know what in the world to do with my situation!

EVALUATION

Post Trauma

Rose has been exposed to and threatened with death. She has experienced bodily injury, emotional and verbal abuse and sexual violence. She has been directly and indirectly traumatized. She has subconsciously absorbed traumatic events which are manifested in reoccurring dreams. Rose has witnessed violence happen to family members and others.

Rose's efforts to avoid external reminders (people, conversations, activities, situations) that bring back the memories, thoughts or feelings associated with the trauma have been ineffective. Her thoughts are intrusive, and she is unable to sleep at night.

Depression

Rose exhibits the following symptoms:

Feelings of sadness and hopelessness nearly most of the day, every day.

Insomnia, psychomotor agitation, fatigue, loss of energy and inappropriate guilt.

Anxiety

Rose displays excessive anxiety and worry that occurs most days. Symptoms have been prevalent for at least six months.

Uncontrollable worry, restlessness, feeling on edge, easily fatigued, irritability, muscle tension and sleep disturbance.

Healing Treatment

Narrative Healing

Deep Breathing

SWEA Tree Color Meditation

Physical Activity

PART TWO
Therapy

Session #3

Light from Heaven peered

Fawn looked up with silent tears

Smile began to glow

Therapist

Rose, Tell me about yourself.

Rose

Okay. Let's see. Where do I start?

Therapist

You can start anywhere you like.

Rose

Okay. When my mother came to Florida to live with me, emotional sadness that lay dormant inside of my spirit was uncovered and took over. Ironic as it may seem, we shared the same sadness. Don't get me wrong, I was happy for her to come, but I didn't realize she was going through hell with her husband of almost thirty-three years. That was a blow to the gut that I wasn't prepared to ingest.

My heart opened as I listened to her describe the chain of horrific events of her life. Her stories of three other marriages sort of merged into one because they were similar.

Her voice trembled as she told of how the men who were supposed to have loved her, all but killed her. The details were very graphic and disturbing. She appeared to be numb as she poured out silent hurt and tears of decades of misery. I listened. I knew that she needed to let it out in order to move forward with anything that resembled happiness.

On July 11, 2018, I became my mother's caregiver. Did I see this coming? No! I had just retired in March of the same year; doctors' orders. My doctor told me I was stressed and my blood pressure needed to get under control. She told me it was my time to care for myself. Her advice was for me to take an early retirement. She said, find a way to let go of that job and let social security and your pension work for you. I took her advice. For the next four months, I began to learn how to slow down, breathe and take better care of myself. I didn't realize how exhausted I was and what it entailed to take care of myself correctly. It is amazing how you can be so busy with your life that you are actually missing your life.

Anyway, my mother's current living situation in Rochester, NY had become unbearable. It was not due to her lack of ability to care for herself; it was due to her living in a verbally abusive marriage. Little did I know, she'd been living in that hell for over thirty years. According to her, husband number four had proved to be just as abusive to her as the other husbands. She claimed he never hit her, but I really don't know what to believe.

Okay, I need to take a moment and step out of my head about my mother. You asked about me.

Here's something for you.

When I was a little girl, I was standing on some wooden steps. As I looked out to the sidewalk, I spotted girl twins. They were dressed in beautiful pastel colored summer rompers that tied at the top of their shoulders. My tiny three-year aged eyes rested on what I imagined to be soft and fluffy colored clouds as I touched them with my eyes. For some unknown reason, I thought that these little girls were mine! Somehow, I knew I would always have them and never let them go. I dreamed about the beautiful twin girls in their pretty pastel colored rompers each night, until the dream disappeared from my imagination while going to sleep.

When I look in the mirror of my past life, I see the reflection of my mother.

Of course, there are some differences. First of all, I did not marry four times! I married twice! Second, my first husband, I don't even want to call him my husband, was a mad man and seemed to be proud of it. However, on his flip side, he was highly intelligent and had a gift of talking. When I met him, he was charming, polite and protective. I think somewhere inside of his spirit, he loved me and truly wanted to care for me, but he did not know how. He behaved and treated me the same way the older guys in the street treated their women. For some reason, the brothers thought that a sign of their manhood was to knock their women around and the sisters thought that getting pregnant gave them their grown woman rights.

Wow! That's the best comment I have ever made about him. Am I healed?

I know I'm flipping back and forth, but back to my mother, is that ok?

Therapist

This is your story. Tell it in the manner that suits you!

Rose

Thank you for that. Anyway, my mother spoke openly and with graphic detail about two of her husbands who were extremely physically abusive. Her first husband, my father, was fifteen years older than her.

He was a soldier in the military during WWII. He fought in battle, got wounded and received the Purple Heart. I think he brought the war home with him and took it out on my mother. As a little girl, I remember them fighting and my mother yelling out and crying. I grew to believe that hitting was normal. When my father spanked my sisters and brothers, I felt left out. I thought he did not love me. I associated hitting with love. My imagination was very active as a little girl. I remember fantasizing about one of the main characters from a TV program called *The Whirly Birds*. It was about two helicopter pilots who, in my mind, were handsome. I fantasized about the one I favored most, spanking me. I figured if my father didn't, someone would. The spanking was my reference to love.

My mother's other two husbands were also verbally, physically and emotionally abusive. Maybe she associated love with abuse. She watched her father beat her mother.

Husband number four's abuse remained a secret to me until June 2018. That's when my sister informed me and stated that Ma'Me wanted to leave him. I was taken off guard and went into combat mode when I heard he was mistreating her. They were two months shy of being married for thirty-three years.

I was devastated, disappointed and angry. I actually wanted to choke his ass. Instead, I put on my boots and met my sister in Rochester, NY that next month. I really didn't have much time to think about the situation in a rational manner.

As a result, I found myself getting tossed back into my past abuse.

Rational thoughts were out the window and another person in my head took over.

While I was in an abusive relationship, I prayed that someone would come and rescue me. I had to lift my ass up and rescue myself without any knowledge of how to do it.

When I think back, this is probably why I kept contacting that asshole and getting back with him.

When I met my second husband, he rescued me. He immediately claimed my four children as his own. He was gentle, fearless and had a quiet air about him that I loved and trusted. His face always came with a smile. I thought he had some sort of mental issue because he smiled all the time. His highest compliment to me was when he told me how amazed he was about how well I cared for my children. He knew I had just come out of an abusive relationship.

One day at the beginning of our relationship, we got up and dressed as usual. He still had a smile on his face, but his eyes said differently. He told me to come with him on a run. I asked him where and he stated that it was a surprise. I nearly shitted on myself when I saw him go to the closet and unwrap a sawed off shot gun that was well hidden under blankets and sweaters. All he said was, "Let's go find that n***a who put his hands on you." I am not sure what brought that on, but I came to the conclusion that it was my nightmares and talking in my sleep. We went through Newark looking for him where we thought he would be. Imagine that! He and I, walking through the hood, him with a trench coat on and a sawed off shot gun underneath! My husband, Ab, went to the apartment of one of the abuser's friends. He gave the friend a message to give to the abuser. I am thankful we didn't find him.

I know Ab would have shot and killed him.

There once was a time I wanted to get married again. You know, just to have a companion. But now, in all honesty, I am not sure who I am or what I want. I am afraid for someone to know me. But then I think to myself, *my husband will need to be an amazing man*. I will not allow him to try and change me into someone he wants me to become, judge or betray me.

Then the thought of being with someone dissolves because I don't have a clear picture of what that looks like. It's a terrible feeling to feel empty and lonely. I know that my loneliness has gotten me into plenty of trouble in the past. This is one of the reasons I became motivated to seek out therapy. I'm feeling hopeless and I am tired of repeating the same mistakes. I need someone to talk to who is nonjudgmental and can offer unbiased advice. Most of all, someone who will listen and not tell me how I should feel. I want to be able to express everything I am feeling because I do not know all that I am feeling. All I know is that I wake up unhappy and just want to go back to sleep. I have nightmares and cannot sleep at night. I get anxiety when I'm around certain people and places, and certain sounds create confusion in my head.

The thought of all the shit that's happened to me throughout my life makes me want to just be by myself, even though I don't want to be by myself!

The conversations with my mother have stirred shit up and it cannot be unstirred. I know it's *my* past but damn, I don't want to be in this frame of mind.

Damn!

Therapist

So, we'll learn new ways of how to cope with the stressors, anxiety and depression. Let's look at this as a Divine opportunity for healing and growth. We will get through this, together.

Rose

You make it sound so easy!

I am tucked under a grown women's skirt listening to the heartbeat of every traumatic experience. My heart has lost its rhythm.

Session #4

Green bird flying high

Wingspan covers the ocean

Free and peace in sky

Therapist

Tell me, how did you manage to leave your first relationship?

Rose

Leave! Shit, he's not gone! He's still in my head!

Anyway, I was seventeen with two babies. My daughter was a year and a half, and my son was eight months. They are ten and a half months apart. My whole body, mind and spirit had been raped. I didn't have any fight left, didn't know how and damn sure didn't know anyone to call for help. Well, except for this one time, I did try to call one of my junior high school friends. Her name was Pam. I found her phone number in the phone book. I called her and told her that I was being beat and sexually assaulted. My subconscious plea to her came out in silent tears. She, in her big sister tone and words, tried to convince me to leave and come live with her and her family. Our conversation continued, until I heard footsteps coming up the stairs. My heart began to pound. My abuser turned the knob and snatched the door open. He said, "Who the f*!@ you talking to?" He snatched the phone from my hands and spoke into it. "Who the f*!@ is this?" I couldn't hear Pam, but knowing how high spirited she was, I am certain she cursed him out. I heard him say, "I'm gonna come over there and blow your f*!@ ing head off and I'm gonna blow your kids f*!@ing head off, too!" He slammed the phone down, turned to me and nearly beat the life out of me. Head, face, stomach, back, threw me against the wall and I am certain I died. When I came to, he was gone. My babies were in their shared crib. My daughter was standing, holding on to the railing with an empty bottle in one hand and twisting the side of her hair with the other hand. My son was lying on his back screaming. No one heard our screams. I lifted myself off the floor, wobbled to the crib and lifted my babies out. I caressed them into my body to comfort their cries. After a few minutes of comforting them, my son went to sleep. I placed them back into the crib. Reaching into the cabinet, I lifted out a box of powdered milk. My mind wondered how long I had been on the floor. My babies must be starving. Trembling and pouring the white dry powder into the bottles without it spilling proved to be challenging. Bottles made. Slowly walking to the bedroom, I reached the dresser and picked up a hand mirror. I looked at my face. I did not recognize myself. Looking into a mirror seemed to be a habit for me.

Therapist

Habit, what do you mean?

Rose

Each time he beats me, I look into a mirror.

Therapist

What are you looking for?

Rose

To see who I am. To see what I look like. Looking at my battered face and hoping I'll get the courage to kill him in his sleep, fight back or leave. I didn't know how to fight back. I was scared. I did not know how to leave. My head was not clear and I was in a constant state of shock and fear.

Session #5

Flood roar through forest

Sun walk kept Fawn from drowning

Lived another day

Therapist

Tell me about when you finally left.

Rose

I looked at my babies. A little bit of reality sank in when I realized that without me, my babies wouldn't have anyone. And besides, I was sick and tired of looking at my swollen face and blood red eyes in the mirror. One day, I looked into the mirror and for the first time, I cried for me. I couldn't stop crying.

I was frightened at what I saw. Without knowing what to do, I called my mother. Our conversation was short. She told me she'd send me money to leave. What I didn't know at the time, was that her husband number three was beating her ass. I found out recently that he was also the king of physical violence and abuse. He was also a drug user. Oh, yeah, she told me all the graphic and detailed stories about the abuse, drugs and violence.

Damn, I wanted to stomp his ass!

Anyway, her plan was to send the money to my older sister. My sister lived in a building that sat in front of the building we lived in.

The only thing that separated our buildings were the backyard. I could look out of my kitchen window across the backyard and see into her window. The curtains were drawn but that is how close we lived to each other. My sister was going through her own hell. It is so amazing how when you are going through shit, you think you are the only one. I have discovered, that is so *far* from the truth.

I enjoyed looking in the backyard. There were rose bushes that grew wild throughout. Even though they were not pruned or cared for, they still thrived. They were so red and vibrant.

One day, those red roses came knocking on my door. A young girl named Tammy, brought me a bunch of roses. I am not sure how she got them, because like I said, they were growing wild. The bushes were all bunched together, and I knew the thorns were sharp.

Anyway, I heard a soft knock at the door one afternoon. Without asking who it was, I opened the door. Tammy handed me the bunch of roses and quickly turned and left before I could thank her. I slowly brought the roses to my nose. After taking a deep breath in, the aroma miraculously stimulated me with a spark of happiness that spread a smile across my face. That "stop and smell the roses" saying is true. In that moment, I felt hope.

My mother sent the money through Western Union so that I could get a Greyhound bus ticket. I'd need a ticket for myself and it would cost half price for my daughter. My son didn't need to pay, he would sit on my lap.

October 1972, I grabbed a duffle bag that had been under the bed and pushed against the wall. I'd been slowly and secretly packing. It contained a few of my babies' outfits and mine as well. Birth certificates, other important papers and a couple of rattlers for them to play with.

I would plan a time I knew he would not be there.

He was so damn predictable! And thank God we still had a phone! I had it all planned out.

The day came and I did not dare show any nervousness or act any different than normal. I did not want him to suspect anything.

He finally left. My heart raced. I fought back the thought of him catching me in the act of leaving. If he caught me, I knew he'd kill me.

I stuck to my plan to leave that hell hole behind and to not look back.

After he left, I played it safe. I waited for about an hour before I made the final preparation to leave. I then called a green cab service. The dispatch said it would be about ten minutes. I grabbed my two babies, duffle bag and proceeded to walk through the inside hallway of my sister's building. We would wait inside the entrance until the cab came. My heart was pounding. I was so damn scared. I thought, if he for some reason showed up, I'd scream and fight until one of us would get killed.

I had no intention of leaving my babies without their mother.

The cab came on time. My daughter was eighteen months and my son was eight months. Both of them sat in my lap as the driver drove us to Penn Station, downtown Newark.

I am glad we had an early afternoon bus departure. If he kept to his regular pattern, he would not have returned home until late in the evening.

If it was the weekend, he would not come back until Sunday morning. He's going to have a fit when he sees we're not there.

It's a peculiar thing, when my mother left Florida to escape the abuse of her second husband, she had four children and also took a Greyhound bus! Our lives have so much in common!

Session #6

Wet tears on room floor

Higher Source paint walls calm blue

Peace love spread from brush

Therapist

How are you feeling?

Rose

I'm not sure.

I take that back. I'm terrified.

Therapist

What are you terrified of?

Rose

I'm terrified that I will die before I get a chance to live. Don't get me wrong, I know that I am physically living, but I feel as though there is more to life than the shit I've been through and all the chaos that's roaming in my head.

I do not think about my past with thoughts, but somehow my mood is distorted. It's as if another energy is wilding out inside of me and I don't know what to do. I have enough common sense to know that life can haunt you if you don't do anything about it.

After all, that's why I'm here!

I realize my past does not define me, but it is a part of me.

Let me restate that; it kind of does define me. Not necessarily in a bad way, but in a, *I'm not going to take any shit* kind of way. Also, my past has helped fashion me into the woman I am today. So, in a sense, it has defined me. Does that make sense to you? Or are you going to write me off as a crazy woman?

Therapist

Rose, you are definitely not a crazy woman. And I would like to add, *you* define who you are. You have tremendous strength to have survived such horrific situations. Please continue.

Rose

I feel as though every part of me needs attending to and the only way that I can make that happen is for me to either go on an extended sabbatical in the mountains or on a quiet beach. Alone!

Session #7

Street poles become trees

Free seagulls perch high land locked

Screeching cries all night

Therapist

Tell me about your current situation.

Rose

I feel so sad for my mother. Her complaints of aches and pains saddens my heart. It's like she is a child showing me where it hurts. There is nothing I can do to make her feel better. I take her to the doctor, I get her medication for pain and other issues and I make certain all her needs and wants are met. But she complains about pain all day, every day and about her past abuse. I am overwhelmed. I understand she needs to talk it out. I redirect the topic, walk away and even just shake my head as if I'm listening. The damage to my spirit and mind has already taken place. I want her to be happy. She has had a hard and painful life. She is aging and is having a difficult time embracing the reality of her changing body.

I think sometimes she thinks I am sixteen. She tries to treat me like a child. I get flashbacks to when I was a teen. I do not like when she watches for me to come home after going somewhere, unlocking the door for me as if she was waiting by it .When I leave home, upon returning I'll cut through the back of our residence so she won't see me coming home. I dislike when she tells me to eat and get rest all the time or to put a sweater on when I go outside. This is nerve wrecking! This sets me off inside of my head! I do not like it when anyone tells me what to do! I have had enough of that! If I say something to her in my defense, I may hurt her feelings. It can be something simple like, *"Ma'Me, it's hot outside or we live in Florida."* Her facial expression changes to sadness and disappointment because she considers this talking back. So, I try my best to speak in a loving way because I realize she does not mean any harm. I almost have to revert to a childlike voice. However, it triggers rebellion and anger inside of me.

I wonder if she is trying to control me.

Anyway, sometimes I sink back into that sixteen-year age girl mentality and think negative thoughts. I quickly redirect my thinking. I also use to stay away from the house for hours to avoid uncomfortable conversations. When I am sitting in the same room, she watches me. If I sniffle, she immediately asks if I'm getting sick. Every little move I make draws her attention to me. I finally retreated to my room a few months back. That became a problem. She scolded me and thought I was getting sick. Imagine that! She scolded me because she thought I was getting sick. Oh, and she has scolded me for a number of things before. If I say something, as a grown woman should be able to do, she acts as if she's fainting or having a heart issue. One time she even fell to the bed. I told her I was going to call the ambulance and she quickly recovered. I am no longer the happy person I remember. I am not able to be free.

I feel as though I am sixteen. I know that I am not able to change her, I'm just trying to figure out how to cope with the situation.

In my heart, all I want for her is to be happy and healthy.

I remember her to be a young, proud, quick moving, quick minded woman.

I know that age brings about a change, however, it is so sad for me to see her suffer and physically decline each day. Her body and mind are fragile. She lets out moans and sounds that break my heart.

Between the two of us, we are one big emotional mess taking up the same space.

Therapist

Tell me about the living situation when your mother first came to live with you.

Rose

We were living together in my studio apartment, sharing the same bed. Sounds like a good bonding moment, huh? When I tell folks this they say, "You are so blessed to have your mother living with you."

Right! My life flipped completely upside down.

Upon waking each morning, we hug and say our good mornings. That's the best part of the day.

That is when the good morning *literally* ceases.

She shares horrific stories about her life. They fill up the space in my mind as she spills out the graphic and detailed abuse stories of her life.

At the same time, I'd watch the beautiful sunrise from my twelfth-floor apartment, her traumatic stories would simultaneously dig holes into my spirit. I would politely sit and try desperately to remain in control of my emotions.

The sun would cease to shine, and dark clouds start to gather and fill the entire studio apartment.

One story she shared was when she was three years old; this one wasn't that bad.

She began, *"I lie in bed waiting for my mother to warm the kitchen up so I could get up and help her bake biscuits. I always wanted to help my mother. I also wanted to be near my mother because my daddy was mean and he beat on her all the time. I felt it was my responsibility to take care of my mother, two sisters and two brothers.*

We lived in a big wooden house, built by my grandfather. It had a big fireplace in the front and back rooms of the house. You could see through the entire house standing in the front. Rooms were divided with curtains.

My grandfather, Grandpa Handy Rayam, died before I could meet him. The story goes, he stayed home and took care of the children while grandma Maryann traveled throughout Florida in a horse and buggy with an organ in the back. She gave speeches to the people and taught school. Grandma Maryann had seven sons and one daughter. My father was the youngest of the eight children. Everybody called them the Rayam boys. My father was mean and not nice to my mother. My Grandma Maryann told him he was going to die with his shoes on. My daddy died at age forty-nine, in bed with his shoes on.

When my mama got pregnant with me, my grandma Maryann told my daddy and mama to come live in the house with her. We called it the plantation.

That's what my mama did. My mama had all five of us children there; Nellie, Lizzie, Leon, Woodrow and me. Well she really had six, but one of the twins she had died. My brother Woodrow was a twin.

I hated being out in the heat, picking tobacco and cotton. I had to ride a mule to get water from the well. My mother begged my father not to put me on that mule at such a young age. The mule didn't have a blanket or anything across it to soften the bumps to my behind. My father didn't have any mercy. He always wanted me to be a boy.

My mother named you after her. She named you Gladys and you got your middle name Gale, from your babysitter Ms. Whitehead.

Three generations lived in grandma Maryann's house. I had my first two children in that same house. A midwife delivered my babies. We lived in the country and getting to the doctor was hard. If a doctor did come, he was usually too late and drunk.

My mother's mother name was Nellie Collier. We called her grandma Nellie. Grandma Nellie was married to Clayborn Collier. Grandma Nellie had five children.

My Grandpa Clayborn was a quiet man. My grandma Nellie was a sassy, spitfire little short mean woman."

Therapist

Quite a family history. Continue.

Rose

Yes, I know!

I worry about my mother. I feel a rush of fear when I hear the bang from a draw closing too loudly. My mother fell off the bed to the floor one night. I heard this loud bump coming from her room. Within a split second, I ran to her room and scooped her off the floor. From that point on, I am not able to sleep too well. I am on edge at night. It's hard for me to be totally asleep.

I am afraid I will sleep through her falling off the bed.

She has a favorite song, "In the Upper Room" by Mahilia Jackson. I love that she loves music. She has a beautiful voice! I bought her a turntable record player. I'm happy and sad when she plays music. Happy that she is enjoying the music she denied herself of for decades and sad because they are always songs of sadness.

Therapist

There is something about sad songs that makes a person feel better. Do you have one?

Rose

Yes. "Here Comes the Sun" by Nina Simone.

SESSION #8

Today is sunning

Tomorrow is dawn and dusk

Yesterday was moon

Therapist

Let's talk about you.

Rose

Wow! I got a little sidetracked, didn't I?

Okay! Here goes. Forgive me if I bounce around with me telling you about myself. I guess in a sense, I am telling you about me.

Therapist

That is true. So, let's hear about *Rose,* about your past. Tell me about your childhood. Start wherever you like.

Rose

Okay, I told you about the twins. That was a happy memory. My first memory of sexual abuse happened when I was age five. It involved two boys and their sister. They were between ages ten through thirteen.

They messed with me every day.

Therapist

What do you mean, messed with you?

Rose

You are the therapist! You know what that means!

I suppose you want me to get it out, for the sake of getting it out!

Do you want the clean, respectable version or do you want the nasty version?

Therapist

Speak freely. It's your story to tell. There's no judgement here.

Rose

Tell you what, I'll give you a combination of both versions!

Messed with means, they'd throw me on the bed and the girl would off take my underwear.

No! Pull down with force! When it happened for the first time, I didn't know what was happening.

She directed the two brothers to take turns placing themselves inside of me. No! Forcing their linky dinks inside of me including their hands. I remember crying and the sister held me down. She sat on my chest and covered my mouth with her hand. She'd tell me to shut up!

My voice muffled its way through her hands while the two brothers did poking things to my vagina that hurt.

I couldn't stop crying, so with large hands that squeezed into my sides and lifted my body off the bed, she carried me into the bedroom closet. I remember the darkness and small space in the closet bringing comfort. She slammed the door shut. I sat in dark stillness.

I felt hanging clothes rubbing against my face. Through the darkness, I felt around the floor and touched a piece of soft clothing. I'm not sure what it was, but it was soft. Without much hesitation, it magically reached my face and became my pillow.

Being in a small dark closet brought relief. I'd cried so much, I'm certain I dozed off to sleep. Startled by the turning of the knob and a quick pull from where I sat on the floor, the girl pulled me back to the bed. They repeated the rape of my body. When she flipped me over to my back, I thought it was over, but they did things to my anus.

Therapist

Where were the adults?

Rose

Working, I guess.

My mother and I went there to stay with one of her friends.

She was in the process of leaving my father.

In the middle of the night, I woke up to her shaking and lifting me out of bed. She didn't turn on the light, she had a flashlight. Through the light of the flashlight, I could see that her face was puffy. I could tell she was sad.

My mother didn't say why I had to get up while it was still dark outside, and I knew not to ask. We quietly left our home, leaving from the back door.

I don't remember where my older siblings were.

My father was very abusive to my mother. I'd hear loud thumps, screams and crashing glass at different times of the night. My siblings and I pretended to be asleep. I was the youngest of four. That meant, I was not included in my siblings' secret conversations. They considered me as a baby. To this day, they still consider me as a baby. Being the youngest meant that I got left out of a lot of fun things.

Anyway, when my mother and I left and began our walk to what was a mystery, I didn't ask her about her bruises; but I wanted to.

One time I heard my mother and grandmother talking softly. I'd stretch my ears to listen when I heard soft talk. It seems like everyone wanted to keep things from me, but I heard things anyway.

My grandmother said to my mother. "If he puts his hands on you again, I'm gonna get the law on him." To my five-year-old mind, this translated to *daddy would be in jail and not be around*. I knew what jail was. I couldn't stop crying.

One evening, or it could have been the same evening, I began to cry.

My father asked me, "Why are you crying?" I said, "I heard Grandmother and Ma'Me talking and they said they gonna put you in jail."

After that, my parents fought. It was the worst fight ever. I noticed my mother's swollen face and closed eye. I asked her if she was okay. She told me she was fine.

I have always blamed myself for that fight and their split.

I'm one big tear drop waiting to fall.

Therapist

Do you still blame yourself?

Rose

No.

Session #9

Muddy rippling pond

Dead stench mixing with clean air

Vultures eat dead fish

Therapist

The path to self-discovery and the healing of your mind, body and spirit will take courage and faith. You already have an abundance of both.

You will need to give your attention to recovering, balancing and maintaining a healthy mind, body and spirit.

In the process of you becoming aware of *yourself* and learning ways to circumvent your emotions, you will start to live a life filled with peace, love and light.

Rose

Will I ever be able to find my happiness?

Therapist

What do you think?

Rose

I think this is overwhelming.

I'm exhausted.

I feel as if I am being pulled into so many different directions. I am having a problem believing I can be put back together again.

I suppress my tears. I am afraid that if I cry, I will not be able to stop.

Do you understand what I am saying?

I always have my guard up. Sometimes I just want to disappear.

Therapist

Have you ever thought about harming yourself or someone else?

Rose

No!

I just want to be left alone and away from everyone. I'm tired of thinking! I'm tired of feeling and not feeling! I want to roll my body into a soft blanket, close my eyes and hum myself to sleep.

Did I tell you that when I was a teenager, I ran away from home?

Therapist

Tell me about that.

Rose

I wanted to live my life the way *I* wanted to live my life. I was tired of being told what to do. I did not feel loved or understood. I felt like I was in prison. I was very lonely.

I was unhappy! I could not go anywhere, do anything or have any type of company! I felt like everything I did was not good enough. I never felt loved! There was always something missing.

I learned at a very early age how to stay out of everyone's way.

Once in a while, I'd get in my two older brothers' way and we would fight.

We never told our mother.

Therapist

Why didn't you tell your mother?

Rose

We didn't want to worry her. My bedroom was my safe place. I read books and wrote poetry. I am not sure what happened to my tablet of poems. There was a picture on my wall of a girl in a small rowboat in the middle of the ocean. I stared at that picture, a lot. I really loved that picture.

Therapist

What became of the picture?

Rose

When my abuser.... you know what, his name was Hassain. When Hassain discovered how much I loved that picture he tore it up in front of my eyes. I felt helpless. It was too late to change my mind and go back home. Besides, I or shall I say we, convinced my mother that he and I were doing good.

Anyway, I played my collection of vinyl records of music on my record player, listened to WNJR radio station, the most popular radio station in Newark. Radio host Hal Jackson played the best music. Google him. And no, I did not take any of my records or record player with me when I moved away from home. Muslims didn't listen to music, sing or dance according to him.

Smokey Robinson and the miracles sang me to sleep each night. I also loved the Temptations, Martha and The Vandellas, Isaac Hayes, and The Supremes.

Therapist

Who was your favorite group or singer and song?

Rose

Hmmmm! I think it would have to be The Temptations. Now, I loved Smokey Robinson and the Miracles but with Smokey, I cried too much. He had that effect on me. Like, when he sang "The Tracks of my Tears" or "Baby, Baby, Don't Cry" all I did was cry. The Temptations hit every nerve in your body. All their songs were my favorite, but I think "Ol' Man River" really did a lot to my spirit. They sang that song a cappella. I was able to hear all of their unique voices and the harmony sounded like heaven. But then there was "You're My Everything." There is an entire story about that song. I'll share later.

During those days, every guy on the block thought they could sing like the Temptations. They would serenade everyone within ears reach each night with hours of a cappella songs by the Temptations. They sounded so damn good! All the girls wanted to be with them, if you know what I mean. They were our Temptations, or the closest we'd ever get to the real Temptations, standing on the corner under the streetlight, singing their hearts out.

Every girl claimed one for herself. I had my eye on the one I wanted.

His name was Bernard. He was one of nine children. Thin, dark chocolate and hazel eyes. He wore beautifully colored Alpaca sweaters which coordinated well with his dress slacks and alligator shoes. He sang all of Eddie Kendricks' of the Temptations lead parts. I thought he sounded better and looked better than Kendricks. It was love at first sound.

Our apartment and his family's apartment were on the third floor. They faced each other on opposite sides of the street. Our building was number 76, and the street was 16th Avenue. He lived in building number 73, 16th Avenue, directly across the street.

Next to my building was a dry cleaner and next to his building was a bar. Tall streetlamps sat on each corner that displayed a dim source of light.

Bernard's sister and I were the same age. She and I went to the same Junior High School. One day, on our way to our neighborhood school, West Kinney Junior High, I handed her a note to give to her brother. At that time, I didn't know his name so, I addressed him as *Cupid*. I couldn't sleep that night from wondering what he would think of the message.

The next day when I saw her on our way to school, she handed me a note. He had written me back, addressing me as, *Love*.

Therapist

Look at that smile on your face! Such a beautiful memory!

Rose

I know! And from that day on, we became secret lovers. I always had a smile on my face during that time. I fantasized about him all the time.

When they gathered under the streetlamp in the evenings, I had to sneak into my mother's room to look out the window. That was the only way I could see and hear my Cupid and his group sing. He was the Eddie Kendricks of the group.

The only way we were able to communicate was from passing notes.

On one occasion, his note said, "I have a special song for you tonight."

We sort of synchronized the time that he and his group would sing. He knew my mother was strict and didn't allow her children to look out the front window. My mother thought that if we looked out the front window, it would invite robbers to our home. She also did not allow us to sit on the front stoops. She made us sit on the back porch or go into the backyard.

The only way for me to hear and see my Cupid was to be in her room at a certain time.

I don't remember how I pulled it off, but I managed to have a front window view that evening for a special song, dedicated to me!

The name of their group was the *Mellow Fellows*. As I peered out of the window that evening, I watched the brothers gather.

After a few rounds of warming up, they assembled themselves according to voices; first and second tenor, alto, baritone and bass. There were five of them.

My Cupid looked up at my window. They bowed their heads for a moment and the next thing I heard was, *"You surly most know magic girl, cause you changed my life, it was dull and ordinary but you made it sugar and spice."* My mouth flung open, my heart beat fast and ecstasy captured me. I was more in love with Cupid at that moment than I was yesterday.

They continued to sing, and Cupid's song of love and magic remains with me, to this very day.

Even if my mother allowed me to date, there might have been a problem. He was twenty years and I was fourteen.

The only choice we had was to keep our secret a secret.

Our secret love grew. We continued to write love letters, he dedicated songs to me while singing under the streetlamp, an occasional hand kiss and subtle eye contact. We had a third-floor romance under the streetlamp on 16th Avenue. I'll never forget!

Therapist

How long did your secret love relationship last?

Rose

It abruptly ended when I met a bad boy. Us girls, liked bad boys!

Therapist

Bad boys?

Rose

Yes! Bad boys! This other boy was a tough ass, bad boy; that was the word on the street.

In order to survive on the street, you needed to be connected with a tough ass group, have a bunch of hard-core brothers and sisters or a kick ass boyfriend. Well, in my case I wasn't connected to anyone. I had siblings, but they were not hard-core. So, I sought out a kick ass boyfriend. I found one that I thought fit the characteristics of what I wanted.

He was a couple of years older than me. I was fifteen and he was seventeen.

I knew his sister. She went to West Kinney as well. Her bad reputation preceded her, just as her brother's. We spoke in passing. Her family lived around the corner on Littleton Avenue, between Springfield and 16th Avenue.

On our way home from school, we'd see each other. She'd be walking with her tough girl group and I'd be walking, well pretty much by myself. One day, I asked her about her brother. She looked at me smiling and said, "You like my brother." I smiled back and replied, "I'm not sure, but he's good looking." That was the end of that conversation.

A couple of days later, on my way to school he caught up to me and said, "I heard you been asking about me." I got quiet. He started talking and never stopped. He told me he had nine brothers and sisters and that he was the oldest boy. His conversation grew more interesting when he boasted about his recent stay at the Youth House. I thought to myself, *"I struck gold with this one, he had been to the notorious Youth House."* Anyone who had been there and survived were looked upon as a bad ass. In my head, I thought, *"This is the one for me."*

Therapist

What made you choose him over Cupid?

Rose

Cupid was too old for me. He had finished school and was working in New York. Also, I knew the new guy would be able to protect me if anyone tried to jump me. People would think twice if they wanted to jump me because I would be connected to him.

During our first conversation while still walking, he told me he was a Muslim.

I didn't know what he meant. "What's a Muslim?" I asked. It was at that moment he gained my full attention. He began to explain Islam to me.

I later discovered it was his own, homemade version.

He talked, I listened. He mainly told me about the MGT, Muslim Girl Training. I didn't know then, but I know now, that his version was toxic, misleading, chauvinistic, domineering and justified physical abuse. He always followed up with a quote from the Holy Quran.

Hassain was his street name. He claimed me as his girl. I felt special and protected. He told me that in order for me to be his girl, I had to stop eating swine, wear longs skirts and cover my head. I would need to learn the Islamic Student Enrollment and Actual Facts. Most of all, he stated, the brothers are in charge. He said, "We are known as the FOI, the Fruit of Islam. You can be my girl, but you have to submit to

Allah." I didn't understand any of it. However, I did every damn thing he told me to do. He spoke with such confidence and intelligence.

Therapist

And Cupid?

Rose

Everyone knew everyone in our 'hood'. Of course, Cupid found out that Hassain and I were talking. Cupid still sang songs with his group under the streetlamp, but we stopped writing love letters.

On one occasion, Cupid made it a point to see me. I had a little part time job in my cousin's corner store for a couple of hours on Sunday afternoons. He knew I worked there, but this was the first time he came in to see me. In my heart, I knew he wanted to keep his distance because of our age difference.

Anyway, he walked in and faced me. Eye to eye, he said, "Hassain is trouble. You are a sweet sister and you know that you are my Love. You will always be my Love."

Before I could respond, he was out the door. The letters stopped but the songs underneath the streetlamp continued. Cupid and Love, forever.

A few years later, Cupid overdosed on Heroin. Heroin ran rampant in our neighborhood and across Newark and the surrounding cities. People in Newark wanted to move to the Oranges, East Orange, West Orange and South Orange, to try and escape the killer, *Dope*. However, it was just as prevalent in those cities as Newark. In our city, we were more compacted in close quarters. So, of course it killed more of us and it was very noticeably talked about, but nothing was done about it. Brothers and sisters just started dying from the Dope on the street.

At age sixteen, I left home to live with my new boyfriend with the hopes of living a happy life.

My mother didn't know what to do with me anymore and our verbal combat became increasingly exhausting for both of us.

My stomach curdled knowing I was hurting her. Her face was always sad. I wanted to change my mind, but I was in too deep. Besides, Hassain wouldn't let me back out of the relationship. I actually tried. I told him my mother didn't allow me to date. He simply told me what to say to her and how to say it. He turned me against my mother, and I didn't know what to do or who to talk to. I felt I was being pulled in two directions and he was winning. This was the main reason for me running away from home, before I finally left home.

She disliked Hassain with a passion but was unable to sway me away from him.

With hurt and frustration, she finally gave in and gave me the go ahead to leave.

I think one of the factors that played a part in her decision was when she found out I was pregnant. I'd gotten pregnant on purpose during a hot summer's day in July.

One day, instead of attending my summer school class, Hassain made the decision for me to come over his cousin's house. He convinced me that getting pregnant was the right thing to do to show her I was a woman.

I was scared and also a virgin, but I was more afraid of him. I remember thinking that my decision to have sex was a mistake. When it happened, there was nothing enjoyable about it. He got angry because I tensed my body. He was forceful and didn't care about my concerns. The only result in the experience was that I became pregnant.

It was too late to change my mind, I recall thinking. During this time, his attitude in aggression escalated. He began to slap me in my face on a regular basis. It didn't matter that I was pregnant. He told me he did this because he loved me. I actually believed him. I had heard the same words come from my father's mouth when he beat my brothers and sisters. So, to me this was love.

Each day, my life became more increasingly a living hell.

One night I dreamed that someone loved me.

Session #10

Moon heart on fire

Ocean tide smothers red flame

Hot embers turn cool

"*Over the course of my life, I have moved across the state of Florida five times.*

I am currently running from my true feelings because they are lost. Looking at them requires me to be in a quiet place of forgiveness and to set my attention on what is going on inside of me. I feel as though I am unable to do that because I am emotionally distracted. I have lapsed into an unhealthy space. The light, my light, is dim. I am struggling to see through the dark thoughts of hopelessness."

SESSION #11

Cinnamon raisins

Ma'Me in blue duster gown

I love you Ma'Me

Therapist

Tell me something about your childhood.

Rose

As a child, I had to learn how to stay out of the way of other family members.

Everyone was older, until my baby brother came along. He is six years younger than I.

Learning how to entertain myself was fun. It involved nature, empty soda bottles, rocks and colorful quilt swatches. I created a world of colorful things to play with.

My siblings ignored me, so I'd sit in a corner and play and talk with my make-believe world of dolls, mountains and trees. By the way, talking to my make-believe dolls that were made from soda bottles and corn silk, gave me the label of always talking. I would talk to them all the time and didn't care whether anyone heard me, or not.

The one thing I couldn't understand was that I was told that my mouth would get me in trouble. When I got older and thought about that repeated statement, I suppose it proved to be true. I didn't know it at that time; I was a child. My teachers beat me in my hand with a thick strip of tire for talking, almost every day. Many of the teachers were mean and hateful.

Therapist

How did you and your siblings get along?

Rose

Like I said, they ignored me. Not necessarily in a bad way. They were caught up in their own private world, I just wasn't a part of it.

One day, I received some unwanted attention from one of my brothers.

Wilbur, my fluffy, soft, chocolate teddy bear, became missing.

I don't remember when Wilbur came into my life, all I know is that he was my best friend!

He slept with me at night and stayed in my bed during the day. I'd snuggle with him at night and during my nap time. I didn't like being in the dark at night, but with Wilbur next to me, the fear disappeared. It was because of what happened to Wilbur that I discovered a new meaning for a Chinaberry Tree that sat in front of my grandmother's house.

The tall green towering tree displayed strong branches, green leaves and round green berries that stunk so bad, you would almost vomit.

My brother next to me in age, took my Wilbur off my bed. This was where I kept Wilbur during the times I didn't have him. My brother went to either the outside pump or indoor water bucket and drenched my chocolate bear with water. He then took him into the field in the back of our house and buried him. When I finally found out what happened, it was too late. Wilbur was covered with mud and unrecognizable. He'd buried Wilbur in the dirt!

I couldn't stop crying. My mother was still at work, so I didn't have anyone to cry to. I threw Wilbur to the ground and ran as fast as I could away from my brother and an unrecognizable bear. I'm not sure how but I ended up in the Chinaberry Tree. I climbed myself onto the highest branch that I could reach. My legs and arms wrapped around one of the strong branches.

Time passed and no one looked for me or noticed I was missing.

When my mother came home, I'm certain she dealt with my brother; I just don't remember.

The tree became my safe place. I'd always climb it when I wanted to get away from being ignored. Climbing up and hanging onto the branches of that tree became my favorite way to pass time.

Damn! I haven't thought about that in a long time!

NOW I'm angry! I feel my head is about to explode!

I would like to scream! Permission to scream!

Therapist

Scream.

Rose

E-Yahhhhhhhhhhhhhhh-Yahhhhhhhhhhhh-Yahhhhhhhhhhhhhhh!!!!

That's better.

Therapist

Take a deep breath.

Rose

They didn't care for me when I was growing up and they don't care for me now! That's how I feel. I have learned to live with it. They don't seem to know how to help or they are so wrapped up into their world. I was wrapped up in my own world, as well.

Therapist

What do you mean?

Rose

March 2018, after being diagnosed with stress and fatigue. My physician *ordered* me to take the remaining of the school year off. Actually, she had me think about the idea of retirement.

I decided to retire in March.

I was thankful to finally get an opportunity to self-care and heal the traumas that were still roaming in my spirit. I'd never had an opportunity to focus solely on me. I must admit, I was extremely tired, but knew how to work on automatic.

It seemed as if I needed permission to stop working and to actually hear the words, "You need to spend the rest of your life taking care of yourself better." I heard her words sing in my head.

Everything in my life began to brighten up.

It's weird how I needed permission to take care of myself.

Each morning became a pleasant renewal of love for myself as I watched the sunrise. I began to bake a lot of healthy organic cakes, I went for long walks, hung out on the beach, started a Mediterranean diet, created beautiful art, began taking Tai Chi classes again and a social life was on the horizon. For the first time, it was all about me and it felt good!

No getting up in the morning for work, I could lie in bed all day if I wanted to and didn't need to explain it to anyone. Walk around the house butt naked and feel good about it.

I was living a simple and happy life!

I could see my children and grandchildren on a regular basis. My grandson and I were beginning to spend more quality time together. We especially enjoyed hanging out at the beach and playing in the sand. Feeling happy felt good!

I finally convinced myself that after decades of teaching high school and raising my children, that I earned the pleasure of caring and spoiling myself with the simple things.

Therapist

It sounds like you were having a great experience. Continue.

Rose

June 2018, I received a phone call from my older sister. She is six years older. I was shocked when she told me that my mother was living in an emotionally abusive relationship and wanted out!

Her husband of 33 years had beat her down emotionally. She waited on him hand and foot for all those years with no appreciation. It wore her body down. All of this was going on and she kept it a secret from her children. When I found out, my mind snapped back to my days of domestic violence.

I was the sibling selected for her to come live with me. I readily agreed.

The only problem was, I was mentally tapped out and was living in a studio apartment in a 55+ community. I didn't think about that. I acted on pure emotions.

Therapist

Were your sister or brothers an option?

Rose

Well, I'm not sure I remember a discussion about her being an option. I do know she had more physical space. I simply don't remember. It seems like part of my brain went somewhere else. I'm guessing my willingness outweighed everything and anyone else when deciding who would take care of my mother. That's my mother and there was no way I could say no.

It's just that I feel some kind of way that no one else was even *considered*. It probably would have still been me caring for her, but at least I'd feel a little better. Damn!

My sister has been through a lot, too. I wish we were closer. When I was eight, my mother sent her to New Jersey to live with our aunt. She went through her own hell while living there.

God knows she has gone through a lot of shit in her life, different shit but same stressors and trauma. We never had a chance to get to really know each other. She calls my mother every day and talks for a long time. That is a huge help. Outside of my sister calling, no one else does anything substantial. One of my brothers lives in the same city and calls her once in a while. It hurts my mother that he doesn't come around. I hear and see the hurt. She will say things I won't repeat. It was her dream to be around her children and grands at this stage in her life. So far, I am the only child that sees her because we live together. My sister visited on Mother's Day 2019. It's hard for my sister to come. She's on a fixed income.

My daughter and son-in-law visit often. My other children call at least three times a month. My two brothers in Rochester call her periodically. So, it frustrates me. I feel as though I am in this alone, with the exception of my sister and her devotion to making daily phone calls from NJ. I know some of the hell my sister has experienced. I want her to heal from the shit in her life. I just wish we had grown up to be close sisters. It brings me joy to see my daughters interact with each other. They display a sisterhood and bond that is so real and loving.

Therapist

Have you ever asked your brother for help?

Rose

Yes, but I refuse to beg someone to help me take care of *their* own mother. He knows what I am doing. He knows that she is his mother, too. It would be great if he could take her at least once a week to lunch, dinner or a ride, so that I can have some in the house alone time. Once a month would also be great! I feel like I am suffocating!

There is nothing on earth that could have prepared me for this. I take one day at a time. My mother has lived a life of disappointment and abuse. Her life stories and being her caregiver has created additional stress, depression and anxiety to my life. A little help would be great!

Let me go back to the point that I am getting away from.

July 9, 2018, my sister and I met at my mother's home in Rochester, NY. Our plan was to get our ninety-year aged mother away from her mean ass husband.

I was on a roller coaster of raw and mostly angry emotions! Mainly anger as to why in the hell was my strong role model living in a f'*#@d up relationship.

I asked my sister to get to Rochester first; I would need her to help keep me calm. When it came to my mother, I would lose it if I thought or got a whiff of anyone mistreating her. I told my mother I would be wearing my boots! She knew what that meant. It meant I was gonna kick ass!!! My sister took my suggestion and arrived a day ahead of me.

Unfortunately for me, I felt a surge of emotions getting stirred up that I didn't' have any control over. I ignored them and went full speed ahead. Looking back and analyzing my behavior, I realize that I was in in a state of past stress and anxiety involving my domestic violence in the past. I fought for the stability needed to stay focused on the rescuing of my ninety-year aged mother.

When I arrived on July 9th, my sister was already there. She did the packing of clothes, pictures and other keepsakes my mother wanted to bring with her. There was a limit to what she could bring because it had to fit in the trunk and back seat of my mother's car. The next morning, July 10th, I packed the items in the car and my sister made certain that my mother had her important papers. Her husband stood and looked on in shock. I don't think he believed my mother would ever leave. My mother sat in a chair looking like a frightened child with a pitbull standing in front of her. He tried to get her to go out with him. He told her he wanted to give her a *piece of money*. She didn't go. That was a definite NO!

We got up early the next morning, packed the last items in the car, loaded ourselves and I drove us away from her husband and home of thirty-three years. After dropping the car off to a storage facility, we arranged for an Uber to take us to a hotel where we would spend the night.

The next morning, July 11, 2018, my mother and I took a flight to Clearwater, Florida. A couple of hours earlier, my sister had taken an Uber to the train station for her return trip to New Jersey.

My grandson picked us up from the airport after a long and exhausting two plane flight. We arrived in Clearwater Beach late at night. I gave my mother something to sleep in and she slept like a baby. I laid next to her in my full-sized bed. I don't remember ever sleeping in the same bed with my mother. I didn't move all night. When I had to use the bathroom, I slide down the bed. I slept next to the wall. She slept on the outside, which made it easy for her to get out of bed.

I was happy my mother made the choice to leave, but I was so confused. I was able to look at her face and tell she endured years of hurt and suffering. She was an expert at wearing the mask of happiness and singing songs of joy, in the name of God. Now that she was away from the bullshit, all that make-believe happiness and joy would be dispelled. What's that saying, *"The truth will come to the light."* And her truth came to the light.

Four husbands and pure hell from all of them! Her own father was abusive. As a child, she watched her father beat her mother nearly to death. We, as children watched our father beat our mother. We knew that she had two other marriages before number four, but I didn't realize the horror she lived through.

I'm bouncing around a little with this conversation, but this is how it is! This shit is all in my head.

Therapist

That's perfectly alright. It's important you tell your story your way. The order doesn't matter.

Rose

Thank you for that. Did I tell you that my mother told me how husband number three drove her to a park one night and proceeded to continuously bash her head into the dashboard of the car? Yeah, she told me this with graphic details. When she told me this story for the first time, a part of me died inside. This story was the tip of the iceberg. She told me about sexual assaults and tons of stories on how my father beat her. She even told me how she stood in the middle of her mother and father when they fought. Her father did not distinguish between her or her mother. My mother would get hit and thrown into the wall. She told me stories of how her father would drag her mother into the woods and nearly beat the life out of her. She'd hear and see her mother moaning and dragging back to the house. She'd run out to help her mother. My mother looks into the distance as she tells this particular story. She said her mother stated, *"Don't let your father kill me."* They lived in the country with no other families around. He could have easily killed her mother. This was during the early thirties.

What breaks my heart is that the very thing she hated and tried to run away from is the very thing she kept running into. I think that her secrets of abuse killed her.

The tiny studio apartment was now an intensive care space. She needed to be treated for years of abuse. I knew I had to keep a close eye on her. My mother and I slept in the same bed, ate at the same table and looked at the same rising sun each morning through our twelfth-floor window.

While lying in bed, she'd share every abusive story with me. From the time we got up and performed our ritual of coffee drinking until the time we lie our bodies down to sleep. I waited on her hand and foot. She was worn out and hanging by thin withered threads.

Ninety years of abuse did all but kill her. As fragile as she is, she is still remarkably strong. God put something in her that caused her to withstand the greatest abuse I have ever heard in my life! I had to figure out a way to listen to her without it causing too much trauma to my emotions. Her being able to openly and freely let out her pain and hurt would add years to her life. Also, it would be the first time in her life that she could breathe and move about from moment to moment without feeling tense or inhibited. She needed to tell her story.

Therapist

That was a tremendous emotional load for you, did you consider therapy, *for her?*

Rose

Yes, therapy was considered. However, she is from a school of thought where you don't talk your business to strangers. Hell, she kept it a secret from her children and friends. She would never be able to pour out her emotions and allow herself to be vulnerable. She has always prided herself with being strong. She was a *rock* for other people. I became her rock.

So, I sat quietly and listened as I cried inside.

Listening to her caused me to always be sad; everyday! Even to this day I am sad. I go to sleep with sadness and wake up to sadness. I am afraid to ask her how she feels. If I do, she will always talk about aches, pains, death and dying. So, I rarely ask. When I do, I try and quickly redirect the conversation with thankfulness of being alive and able to drink a cup of coffee. I have rehearsed lines and phrases that are ready for when I need them.

Hopelessness has taken over.

Therapist

How has hopelessness taken over?

Rose

There is no light at the end of this tunnel. If there is, I am unable to see or sense it.

I do not believe anyone is capable of understanding my mother's past or capable of caring for her in a loving, compassionate and empathetic manner. With me knowing this, I know that I am in it for the long haul. However, each day becomes increasingly harder. I am witnessing her body, mind and spirt decline. And I am sick and tired of people telling me, I am blessed and lucky to have my mother still alive and in my life! Hell, I know that! They, with their narrow tunnel vision, do not know what is behind the scenes. They have not lived my traumatic life! They have not heard my mother's traumatic stories! They do not understand the destruction of my mind, spirit and emotions to hear and see your role model being transformed into something unrecognizable. Hell, I wonder and question why in the world she kept falling for the bull shit from men! Why in the hell did she suffer in silence for so many damn years! Am I really like her, as so many people say? She thinks I am walking in her shoes! Those shoes do not fit my feet.

I feel I am in a hopeless situation because there is no out for me. For the rest of my life I will carry this traumatic emotional weight.

If she finds out that I am depressed or suspects that she has added to my stress, she would not forgive herself.

We would start to walk around each other, feeling uncomfortable. So, I keep a smile on my face, say "yes ma'am, no ma'am," so that my mother can live happy for the rest of her life.

Damn, my life is totally wrapped up into her life, in more ways than one.

I am feeling… at this moment, I don't know what I am feeling!

I am angry! Anger and tears do not mix.

Therapist

Just for this moment, stop and breathe.

Session #12

Flying against wind

Black bird struggles across sky

Cry alone up high.

Rose

Every time I go to a doctor appointment, they always ask, *"What physical diseases run in your family?*

Do either of your parents or grandparents have heart problems, hypertension, diabetes....?"

I want to say, *"Hell yeah, all of the above."*

They never ask, *"Have either of your parents ever suffered from post-traumatic stress, have they ever been sexually assaulted, were they abused as children or have they ever nearly starved to death?"*

Correct me if I'm wrong, but I think it's equally important to find out about mental health issues with the same intensity as finding out about the physical health issues. I truly believe a lot of the physical diseases are symptoms of mental diseases. I have high blood pressure and I know it's stress related.

Based on some of the stories I've heard about my family, depression, domestic violence, and sexual abuse are on the list of mental health issues. In my family, there has been at least four generations of alcoholics. My great grandmother had two sons who died from the disease. My grandmother had one son who died and a daughter who is an alcoholic. There was also depression and PTSD among my grandmother's children. PTSD was not on the table of mental illness, so of course it went untreated.

She had two sons who fought in and survived the Korean War. They actually fought three wars. The first war was the actual combat against the so-called enemy, the second was racism while in the military, and the third being the war of racism and discrimination once they returned home. They brought the war home with them and tried to escape using alcohol and isolation. Within my mother's children, I have abused drugs and alcohol, suffered from depression, domestic violence and sexual abuse. Oh, and racism and discrimination. Damn, I inherited everything! My children, well I have two sons that I have not seen or heard from since 2005. That speaks volumes without saying anything.

Facts do not disappear in the dark.

Session #13 (Sons)

Silk flowing river

Unearthing rocks in my heart

The sun is shining.

Therapist

What's on your mind, Rose?

Rose

My four sons.

Therapist

What about them?

Rose

I am having a difficult time dealing with the fact that three of my four sons are not in my life. The first two chose not to and my third son is incarcerated. Tehuti and Sebek are the spiritual names I have given to my two older sons. The names are Kemetic. Tehuti, my oldest, is a wise old man who gives advice. Sebek is very intelligent and verbally expressive. My third son is Herukhuti. He is strong, fearless and values truth.

My fourth son is Heru. Heru is protective, a great provider and his heart is close with his mother.

They don't know that I call them those names; well the two youngest sons know.

Therapist

What comes to mind about your sons?

Rose

I often think about what I could have done differently while raising them. I try to trace back how I treated them and the type of relationship we had. I am trying to understand why the older two have cut me out of their lives. I am lost for answers.

My fourth son talks about and remembers his childhood. His stories are filled with love and memories. The only hard question he ever had for me was, *why didn't his father play more of an active role in his life?* I told him that was a conversation for him and his father.

I just miss my sons and I'm sick of people telling me, *"It's not your fault they turned out like that."* That's a bunch of bullshit. Who the *hell* are they to tell me how to feel about my *own* sons! A parent will always feel as if they could have done something differently. And regardless to what our children do, we still love them.

If any parent says differently, they are lying!

I don't let the thought consume me, but I will always wish the *impossible*, that I could do it over and better.

Therapist

Realize that the life your children lived are the lessons that will help them to become healthy and balanced men and women. There was no wrong or right way. It was the only way you knew at that time in your life. You had more insight than you give yourself credit for. Your first child at sixteen and living in an abusive relationship. You had so much courage to live and survive that! Your sons will eventually see their mother, but I do believe they love their mother.

Rose

Thanks for that! But I had my children when I was too young! My first son at age seven-teen, second at nine-teen, third at twenty-two and fourth at thirty-two.

I believe being a certain age and living under certain conditions does make a difference in how you raise your children.

Therapist

What do you mean?

Rose

I was young and clueless on how to raise children. All I knew how to do was what I did. I feel guilty that I couldn't do more or give them more. For some reason, I feel my sons suffered more.

Therapist

Suffered? What do you mean by, *suffered?*

Rose

I think some of my sons may have felt neglected, emotionally abandoned, and angry. Now that I am an older woman, I have given it plenty of thought. I also think that someone may have hurt them either physically or sexually without my knowledge. I feel in my heart that they silently called for their Ma'Me, but I didn't hear them.

Therapist

How did you come to that conclusion about your sons?

Rose

Because, one of my daughter's shared a story with me about herself that brought me to tears. It was a story that happened to her which involved a couple of my sons and other older people who harmed them. Her story forced me to reflect on as many details about my children growing up as possible. Even the smallest detail, like why my oldest daughter slept in clothes every night, why my oldest son played a song by Metallica entitled "Kill My Mother Tonight" and why my third son turned to the street.

My heart is heavy with hurt at the thought of someone doing the same things to my children that were done to me. I have to pray hard for silence in my head, that it doesn't destroy me.

I was always on the go. I took care of food, clothing, shelter and gave them plenty of love, hugs and kisses. I made sure they attended school every day, tried to keep them engaged with fun things, I worked at a fast food restaurant at night, went to college, abused drugs and had men friends in my life. I cared for and loved my children. I feel as though I was *blind* to a lot of what was going on right in front of my eyes.

Therapist

You coped and navigated through your life the best way you knew how. Your subconscious may have blocked certain things that happened because of what you went through. When certain trauma happens in a person's life, they can block it out entirely until it's triggered. One of your coping mechanisms were for you to block out a lot of what was going on around you. It didn't mean you didn't love or care for your children. It meant that, in order for you to survive the post trauma, you withdrew and became *blind* to certain instances in order to survive.

I call it the *"roaches on the wall syndrome."*

Rose

Roaches on the wall! What are you talking about?

Therapist

I grew up in an apartment building where everyone had roaches. When we went to bed at night, we naturally turned the lights off. When we turned the lights on to go to the bathroom, the roaches on the wall would scatter and run back to their cracks in the wall. No matter how much Raid Roach Spray we used, the roaches would still come back. We got to the point where when we turned the light on, we stopped seeing the roaches. We had to stop seeing the roaches in order to go back to sleep and get a good night's rest.

Rose

Wow! That's so interesting. So, you're telling me that my past trauma created a sort of blindness to what was going on with my children?

Therapist

Yes. You were mentally and spiritually unavailable to see what was right before you. That's not a bad or a good thing. You experienced physical and sexual trauma in the past. That being the case, an unconscious *wall of blindness,* stood between the reality of what was taking place, as it relates to the trauma, in your children's life. There is a strong possibility that had that wall not been there, you could have endured a mental breakdown rendering you incapable of caring for your children. So, essentially your so-called blindness to certain instances allowed you to care for your children in the only way you knew how. It saved your life as well as theirs.

What's courageous and great is that you are tearing down the wall and getting rid of the roaches.

Rose

Thank you for that.

I am certain my children are holding on to my and their hurt and pain. That bothers me.

My daughters hold a lot in. My sons let it out. My two oldest sons' anger have been directed at me and in their adult relationships with women. The two of them have been verbally and physically abusive towards their partners.

Damn, I wish we could have had family counseling. I really want us to uncover and let go of our painful past. I wish all of us, daughters and sons, could form a circle of love and heal together. I really believe my children experienced some of the same hell I experienced as a child. Also, their world revolved around my world.

The last time I laid eyes on my two eldest sons was in the summer of 2005.

I know the state my oldest son lives in and I know that he knows how to contact me. I don't know how to contact him. I think one day I will hire a private detective so I can find both of them. Looking on my own hasn't worked.

Again, I get tired of people saying, *"They will get in touch with you when they are ready."*

But then I think, what if they reject me? What if they say mean and cruel things to me? Will I be able to recover? It's sort of like my third son being in prison. As of date, I have not been able to go visit him. He has been locked up since 2015. I have tried to gather the courage to go visit, but each time, I literally freeze up and start to get some sort of stomach issues. My mind shuts down and I am unable to gain enough composure to make it to the prison. When he first got locked up, I had a nervous breakdown. I collapsed to the floor and remained there for hours. My immune system was compromised, and I contracted Vitiligo. Our entire family took a hard hit when my Herukhuti got locked up.

Anyway, I realize that my sons are not ready to face me. When they face me, they will realize that we are the same.

My oldest son is my second child. He is much like me in so many ways. He has always been creative and poetic. My Tehuti is wise before his time and is also a good listener. He has a true renaissance spirit.

I remember one day, he was sitting quietly in our kitchen at the table. He had to be about ten or eleven. As I was passing, I glimpsed a bewildered expression across his face. I asked him, *"What's the matter?"* He said, *"I don't think I can draw anymore."*

"What do you mean?" I asked as I stopped in my tracks. He replied, *"It's been a long time and I don't think I can do it. Everything I draw turns out wrong."* I told him to *"Sit tight."* I walked over to my bookshelf and pulled out an African History picture book. It contained beautiful colorful pictures. I flipped through it until I found the right one. I walked back to the table and sat down. I felt his eyes asking, *"What is my mother doing?"* I placed the book in front of him and showed a picture of a beautiful chocolate African girl. Her head was bald, and she wore a thin band of colorful beads around it to represent her crown. The girl's bright, happy eyes sparkled. Draped across her shoulders was a brightly colored fabric shawl of red, gold and green. His eyes were planted on the beautiful girl. Underneath her picture was her name, Uzuri! He asked me, *"How do you pronounce that and what does it mean?"*

"U- zu- ree, and it means beautiful!" I replied. *"Now, this is a picture, I know you can draw."*

I left him at the table with a pencil, a large 10x11 sketch pad and a pencil sharpener.

When he finished, it was perfect! My heart melted. I said to him, *"I knew you could do it."* He smiled at me and said, *"Ma'Me, this is for you."*

I framed the picture in red transparent cellophane paper. The beautiful Uzuri hung on the wall in our front room and every front room thereafter. Around 2005, the picture and a lot of my belongings got left in storage. I would do almost anything to get that picture back. The good thing is, I'm left with the memory of watching my son draw it and the happiness it brought him when he realized he still had *the touch.*

The last time I saw my Tehuti was in 2005. He came to visit when I lived in Tallahassee. It was a beautiful visit. Six of his siblings had relocated to Tallahassee, so we were able to gather as a family. The only child that was missing was Herukhuti. He was still in New Jersey. My Tehuti was extremely loving and supportive.

Tehuti named his first-born daughter, Uzuri. So, I know that we share the same memory.

He'd driven all the way from New Jersey to see me. His older sister called and told him that I was going through chemical therapy.

The next thing I knew, he was pulling up into the parking lot in a brand-new Jeep Cherokee.

We spent days of quality time. I enjoyed the time and our conversations we had. I took him to my favorite get-away, St. George Island. He bought me a grey t-shirt with a turtle on it. He bought a beige one for himself.

His last words I recall him saying remains in my heart and mind. He said, *"Ma'Me, do what makes you happy!"* Such a simple statement, but no one had ever told me that before. I try and strive each day of my life to live true to those words. Here lately, it has been a struggle.

I still feel the impact of his words and the love that fueled them.

My son, you asked Heaven to send you so that I would learn that I deserve to be happy. Before you said those words to me, I had never thought of what made me happy. Thank you for your words of wisdom and being my first-born son. Your creativity is sealed into my heart and connects with your heart. There aren't any words, just musical notes, dance, and the gift of telepathic vibrations. Without you, I would not wonder about happiness.

My son was born at Martland Medical Center, Newark, NJ.

"Do What Makes You Happy"

Therapist

What do you want to say to your sons?

Rose

I don't know.

That's a deep question. Words are meaningless. There is no way I could possibly express the decades of rehearsed conversations that lie dormant in my heart.

I want to hug him! I want to simply say, 'I love you my son. I have always loved you and held you and nothing will ever change that. You are my son!"

My second son, and third child, Sebek and I have always had a great relationship. When he was a baby, his smile filled the room. He had always been swift with his movement and clever with his words. He is the son that always wanted to make sure the family had cleaning products and chicken. On the weekends, he'd get up and go bag groceries at Montana Meats, on Central Avenue in East Orange. The grocery store was a block away from our home. He'd leave around 7:00am to beat the rush of young boys trying to compete for the same bagging job. He was always successful. Everyone on the block knew my children and so did the manager of Montana Meats. I think he favored my son. My Sebek had a charm and was very articulate.

Besides, folks knew I'd hurt them if they bothered my children. We lived at 32 South Munn Avenue. It was a pretty nice neighborhood during that time. The library was on the corner and Memorial park was around the corner. The police department was a little further down across Main Street. On Central Avenue was East Orange General Hospital. Our building sat between two major streets, Central Avenue and Main Street.

Living in East Orange on Munn brought my children and I closer together. We were able to breathe a little better. Living conditions changed for the better. We no longer had to live in conditions that were depressing. I was able to move us from a one room basement apartment, sleeping on mattresses on the floor, to a two-bedroom apartment, sleeping on bunk beds. Our family became one with the people on the block and the businesses looked out for the children. We were a thriving community. Yes, we did have our share of problems, but we always worked them out.

Anyway, my Sebek would bag groceries from about eight in the morning until about noon. He would come home with bags of groceries. Chicken, milk, eggs and lots of cleansers. I think he was a germaphobe.

One day, there was a flea market being held at a church on our block. Of course, my Sebek went! He came back home with two wooden statues. He said, *"Ma'Me, this is for you."* I hugged him and cried silent tears of love. I still have one of the statues to this day.

Also, when he was a little boy, his favorite book was, *I Wonder as I Wander* by Langston Hughes. I'd read to him every night. He required that! He'd also read to me.

He named his first child, Langston! I know that he remembers and holds that memory as a treasure in his heart; as do I. He is my son that is gifted with verbal expression and communication.

My Sebek suffered a great lost. He lost his wife during delivery of their third child. I don't care to go into any details.

I don't know where he is, but I am certain he knows where I am. I pray he wants to see me.

Thank you, my son, for choosing me as your mother. You are a gift from Heaven. Through you, I am in love with poetry and prayer. Your rhythmic voice filled my head and heart with love and wiped away unwanted and unnoticed pain. I was able to uncover expressions of myself and find my voice. Without you, that would not have been possible. Your birth was the gift of expression and communication. God knew I needed a happy spirit from heaven to always smile and speak words of love. I hear you my son.

My son was born in St. Mary's Hospital, Rochester, NY.

"I Wonder as I Wander"

Therapist

You may not be able to see or understand the dynamics that are taking place with your sons or yourself. But here is something that is worth understanding. Your sons are in the process of growing, healing and learning how to live with past trauma, just as you are. It may take time for them to face certain realities and to ground themselves in the truth of who they are and why they are the men they have become. And in turn, it is taking time for you. Fortunately, you reached out for help. Who knows, they could be receiving help, as well.

Rose

I'll hold on to that. That's a ray of hope!

Therapist

Please continue. I know you have four sons, that's only two.

Rose

My third son and fifth child, Herukhuti! Ride or Die!

I met his father at age twenty and we were inseparable. Ab, which is what I called him, came to be my second husband. He claimed my four children as his own, unconditionally. He still holds that claim. I got pregnant within a couple of months of us getting together. My youngest, at that time, was eighteen months.

I actually experienced a happy pregnancy for the first time. I even had a baby shower. His father made sure we always had a refrigerator filled with food and that my other children had everything they needed.

He is Herukhuti because he is very courageous. My Herukhuti was born in a home filled with love and happiness from two parents. We lived in the Weequahic Towers, located in Newark, NJ. The Towers, during the early 70's, were fabulous. There was an indoor swimming pool, steam sauna, exercise room, a security guard in the lobby to announce visitors, a doctor's office in the lobby and to add fabulous on top of fabulous, the building faced Weequahic Park. Our apartment on the 14th floor overlooked the park. We had hard wood floors and picture windows with a view that overlooked the lake in the park.

Anyway, my Herukhuti weighed 7pounds and 11ounces at birth. He was a cheerful and quiet baby. His calm and pleasant smile spoke happiness.

I remember when he started kindergarten. He and his four older siblings attended an Islamic school in Newark, on South Orange Avenue. The name of the school was Sister Clara Muhammad. They were fortunate to attend such a wonderful school and to also get transportation by a beautiful Muslim family. Their family and ours had children around the same age. Our children became friends with each other. My oldest daughter and their oldest daughter became best friends. Although they have not seen each other in years, they still carry their best friend bond. The family and I are in contact on social media.

So, he was in kindergarten. When the teacher called on him to read, he simply looked at her and smiled. The teachers were old school Islam.

That meant they didn't call me to tell me or other parents about the little things that happened. His teacher, Sister Umakaya, decided to call his sister into the classroom so that she could ask if there was something wrong with him. The sister that went into the classroom to conference with the teacher was two years older than her brother. She told the teacher that he could talk and that nothing was the matter with him. His sister then picked up the assigned reading, sat beside him and told him to read. My Herukhuti read every word in the passage! His reading exceeded the expectations of the teacher. Later, when I found out, his teacher confided in me that out of all her years of teaching, she had never come into a situation like this. She said that it was a life learning lesson for her and to never assume the worst due to the silence of a child. My Herukhuti was a great listener. He absorbed information which placed him at the head of the class. However, my daughter continued to visit his class during reading period.

Herukhuti had lots of talent. He played the violin and played football during high school. He was the son who would test the water of dares, just like his mother. His courage has always placed him in situations and places that the average person would not dare to go. It will be this same courage, after harnessed, that will create and transform a great man. In many instances, his courage is a reflection of my courage. He has always done things his way and would not bend to anyone else's way of thinking.

I recall him losing interest in school and eventually leaving. He went to job corps and did extremely well. He had less than a month left in the program and would graduate with a certification for the program he was in. One of his friends in the corps had a problem with some guys. My son took it upon himself to defend his friend by beating up a couple of the guys at one time. The corps had a zero policy for fighting. They dismissed my son short of a month before completing the program. That's how he is. He is loyal and if he got your back, he got your back. He is a warrior, and has it tattooed across his back.

When he became a teen, Herukhuti took it upon himself to be that son who would kick ass if there was a problem. His brothers and sisters knew that he would go to war for them. I remember when we lived in Tallahassee, Florida and his younger brother, Heru, was in high school, a problem came up. Heru was sixteen and Herukhuti was twenty-six. He had just relocated from Jersey, so that raw Jersey energy was still roaming and pulsating throughout his body. Heru called him and told him that he was going to have a fight after school with some dude and he was certain it wasn't going to be a fair one on one fight. Herukhuti immediately left the house dressed in a "wife beater" t-shirt, a pair of jeans and sneakers. I was at work. He arrived at the school just before dismissal. He told Heru not to mention to anyone of him coming. The fight broke out with just the two of them. Heru was kicking ass; the friends of the dude didn't like that. They proceeded to jump in and with street fighting techniques mixed with wrestling, kick boxing and Kung-Fu, Herukhuti slide through the crowd and put the would be threat to rest. A school security guard began to break up the fight but Herukhuti put his arm across, blocking the guard's effort and said, *"Let them squash this now, or we can come back and do this every damn day until it's over."* The security guard retreated.

That's how he is; quiet, strong, fair and don't take shit! We are very close! He's always saying to me, *"Stop letting your emotions get in the way."* That is his way of saying, *"I can't handle it if I know you are worrying or stressed."*

They say the very thing you run from, usually hits you in the face at some point in your life. For my Herukhuti, it was him going to prison. He knew how it nearly killed me when his father went to prison, so he never wanted to hurt me like that. He knew that would be a deal breaker for my mental sanity. At age nineteen, he went to prison while in New Jersey.

On April 22, 2015, my Herukhuti got shot and went to prison again.

He got caught up in a serious scuffle. My son, who was so good at telling me to not let my emotions cloud my vision, ended up letting his emotions get the best of him for a split second. That split second is all the time it took for him to make a near grave mistake. He got shot and was sentenced thirteen years for a crime.

Yes, I had an emotional breakdown! I have not recovered.

Thank you, my son, for choosing me as your mother. Your presence from Heaven was to show me how determined I needed to be in my life. Also, to help me understand and rely on wisdom instead of emotions. And in the process of it all, loyalty is important. Loyalty stands strong whether we see each other in the flesh or close our eyes and feel the essence of one another's energy. Your presence has showed me what being a true warrior, one who fights to win, is all about. Thank you for choosing me as your mother. Through you, I am determined to do what I must do and not be ruled by my emotions.

My son was born in Beth Israel Hospital, Newark, New Jersey.

"Stop letting your emotions get in the way!"

My fourth-born son is my Heru! His older three brothers are missing in action; action with the family. He has the role as the eldest man within our midst to protect us. It was devastating to watch his expression and feel his pain when his brother, Herukhuti, got locked up.

My fourth son and seventh child Heru was born on a Sunday, Father's Day, 1987. There was thunder, lightning and rain a storm going on while I was in labor. When the thunder came, it brought on a contraction.

My sister-friend, Thelma, was by my side the entire time. We met years ago at a fast food restaurant in Irvington. Both of us worked the night shift at Stuffy's Chicken. We became friends and quickly realized that both of us lived on Munn.

Each time a contraction came, her comforting hands and soothing voice relaxed me. She was from Jamaica and in a thick accent she chanted words that roamed throughout my body.

My son Heru was born to the beat of a symbolic drum as it stormed. According to ancient signs and symbols, this is a spiritual blessing for him. Heru represents a strong will and leadership. Also, he was my seventh child, a very spiritual number. He is referred to as a "mama's boy" by his siblings. It doesn't seem to bother him, and I am glad. All it means is that he'll protect his mother and will not disrespect her.

When he came into the world, he was extremely determined. I had to return to work when he was three weeks old. He didn't like that. I had a trusted sitter who lived in the building. She was a longtime family friend. She told me he cried so much that she thought he was going to hurt himself. I was desperate, I had to work! I came home one evening and heard the same story about his crying. The sitter told me she would give it one more day. That evening, I had a heart to heart, cheek to cheek, tear drop to tear drop conversation with my son. I explained to him how Ma'Me had to work to take care of everyone and that I would always return home. I told him how much I loved and missed him. I asked him to please not cry anymore.

The next day upon picking him up from the sitter, she said to me that he miraculously stopped crying. This is how he was. It seemed that if I explained things to him with heart to heart conversations, he'd understand. He was very perspective and strong willed.

I nursed him, and that was a battle. For some reason, he fought me to not nurse. I attributed it to being at the sitter and sucking on a damn bottle. He nursed a little, but he soon required more, and he selected how that more would be distributed. The bottles won!

He has always, I mean always, had a determined will. If it was something he didn't want to do, he wouldn't do it. I recall him as a toddler at age three, defying his father each time a kufi was placed on his head. He didn't like it on his head and there was nothing anyone could do to get him to keep it on.

When he was in Middle School, a group of boys thought they could jump him. They had the nerve to follow him home. During that time, we were living in Tallahassee, Florida. His Middle School was directly across the street. As I was pulling into the community, I saw a group of children in a circle. I knew what that meant; someone was fighting. As I drove in, I glimpsed into the crowd and saw that it was my son. *Oh, hell no,* I thought.

I pulled in, put my car in park, slung the door open, left my pocketbook inside, didn't close the door and ran into the crowd. Heru was slamming bodies into the ground, as quickly as they tried to charge him! I yelled, "GET THE F*@# OFF MY SON!!!" The crowd dispersed.

Heru dressed extremely well! He was self-employed at age twelve. He washed cars on the weekends. He would receive requests during the week and got it done between Saturday and Sunday. He had one helper.

My Heru had a rap group he formed. The name of the group was Heirs 2 the Throne. They were really good. I helped them rehearse and had as much fun as they did. He organized the rehearsals and wrote a lot of the lyrics. They performed at a few locations. I do believe that if they had a good manager, they would be at the top of the Rap world. The group was diverse, and their fans loved them. His talent was endless. I still have his CD's.

He is the only son that I had the blessing to see graduate from high school. He earned a high school diploma and culinary certifications. He went to his prom and experienced the entire high school graduate experience.

Thank you, my son, for speaking to me with love and kindness. Thank you for letting me experience what it feels like for a mother to see her son graduate from high school. I am grateful for the man that you have become. You chose to be my son so that I could experience what it is like to have a man stick around and not sacrifice his family in place of mundane things. I have learned and experienced faith in myself from the moment of your conception. God knew I needed a seventh birth. You knew you held the heart of faith and chose me for your mother. I am thankful to have given birth to the faith in myself.

My son was born in Beth Israel Hospital, Newark, NJ.

"Heir to the throne?"

My Sons

My sons, you are forever

You gaze into a foreign world with deer stuck eyes

As time gets away from you

I am your heartbeat

If your heart stops, we stop

In search of your father who is a ghost that haunts us as we sleep

Reoccurring dreams transform into conscious thoughts

Awaken into tomorrow wearing the face of alright

Your face is a display of abandonment

As you search for empty memories

Silently wondering what's this heartbeat that I feel

Relentless fangs of Armageddon

Cycles of constant battles perpetuating and dragging out your day

Unconscious actions place you deeper into a hell that ropes your tired spirit captive

Soon we all die and frowning as we welcome death

An illusion exists showing a life that created a smile

Only to become a myth

Warped disfigured and mudded with the stench of forgotten born generations

Like your father and the father before your father

Your inheritance blares a flaming spear

Escaping the torrential calm of a man-less hell

Warriors stand yet still afraid as they fall

An illusion my son

Metamorphosize into the man you are to become

We are not an illusion

I am your heartbeat

You are my son

I love you

Place your hand over your heart

I place my hand over my heart

Feel your Ma'Me

As I feel you my son

Feel my love as we are one.

SESSION #14 (DAUGHTERS)

Sky speckled with stars

Early morning music sings

Lips touch black coffee

Counselor

Tell me about your daughters.

Rose

It was my dream to have a girl first. I wanted to dress her in pretty dresses and put her hair in ponytails with colorful ribbons and barrettes.

On Good Friday, 1971, my dream came true! My first born was a baby girl. She weighed six pounds and was so beautiful. Back then, the baby couldn't stay in your room with you. If you were nursing, they'd bring the baby to you throughout the day and night.

Her little sweet spirit was so gentle and soft. I held her close into my bosom and knew I could never let her go. All of the labor pains disappeared from my memory. The thought of her father and how he treated me faded away. All I could think about was the blessing of having a beautiful baby girl. She was perfect. Throughout the night, I'd go to the nursery window and watch her. On the second night, one of the nurses let me keep her in my room longer than usual. I stayed three days in Martland Medical Center in Newark, NJ. The name of the hospital has changed since then. The hospital is now called, College of Dentistry and Medicine.

My mother came to Jersey from Rochester, NY on the Thursday before I gave birth. It was as if she knew I was about to deliver. On Friday while staying with her sister, I called to tell her I was in labor. She made arrangements with her first cousin to come to my apartment and take me to the hospital. Where was my baby's father? Out in the streets. Actually, he was a coward and did not want to show his face to my mother. He had her child living in abuse and poverty.

Anyway, I don't want to talk about his horrible ass, I'm going to stay on my baby girl's birth.

My mother and her cousin took me to the hospital. I was in labor for a few hours. It didn't hurt or last as long as I imagined.

At 9:12PM, my first baby was born to the world! When the nurse said, "It's a girl," I actually saw stars pour out from my head and fill the room. I laid my eyes on her and shed tears of happiness! Her aura radiated a soft glow of Pink.

The Pink was not because of her body color, it was due to her soft and gentle spirit.

From that moment on, her spirit color became Pink. She was dressed in Pink when I took her home. Her mannerism has always been Pink when she was little. Pink is a soft and gentle color that matched her spirit. I didn't know it at the time, but since then I have learned a lot about colors and our auras. She was definitely Pink. I didn't make her that way, she was born that way.

My little girl was the pink rose quartz in my life. Self-love and the opening of the heart on all levels.

My Pink baby girl grew up to be a beautiful woman. I have always worried about her because she saw so much of my traumatic world. Afterall, I had her when I was sixteen. She has been present every step of the way. Whether she was in my womb or in the same room, she's been there enduring everything I experienced. My internal and external pain and abuse hit her directly and indirectly. I protected her as best as I could. I wasn't conscious to the fact that she was caught up in my hell. I was too busy trying to survive and stay alive. I still worry about her. She carries just as many scars as I carry.

On top of my shit, she has her own shit that is unique to her own life path.

Because she was the oldest, her responsibility in the home was massive! It was not intended to happen like that, however that was what life unfolded for her and I. I depended on her and she knew it. Ever since she came into the world, she wore the look of wanting to protect me.

Her mannerisms were soft, gentle, caring and loving. She knew my soft spots and how to boost my spirits. In the process of her keeping her eyes on me, she took her eyes off herself. My world became increasingly painful and too hard for her to endure. Her Pink began to get murky. I didn't realize this because I was being buried in an abusive hell and taking her with me.

She was the baby for ten and a half months before I had a second child at age seventeen.

By that time, it was too late. She'd seen, heard and suffered too much before she became one year of age.

My daughter became my number one support. We were very much in sync. I didn't have anyone else to depend on, so I depended on her.

Looking back, I wish to God I could have did things differently. I know that my dependence on her was because I didn't have anyone else. She was on the front line of my life with me. The responsibilities included helping with her younger siblings. Within a matter of seven years, there were five siblings under her. Ironing, washing, child sitting and making sure the doors stayed locked when I had to go on errands. The only thing she did not do was cook. I did all the cooking, but she'd make sure her brothers and sisters ate at a certain time.

When I worked at night, she had the night shift. She was around nine when I started college. For the first year and a half, they had a sitter. Then the unthinkable happened. I came home from class one evening and she had a strange look on her face. She ran to me and told me that the sitter had slapped her sister in the face. It was true. That heffa' had put her hands in my child's face. All I remember is that the sitter's mother and father had to intervene. Afterwards, my back was against the wall. We had a family meeting. I explained to them why it was important for me to continue classes and that I didn't have anyone else to watch them. We formed a closer bond. I began to leave them in the evening three times a week. My Pink baby, at age ten, held it down while I worked on getting a bachelor's degree. She made certain they ate, they teamed up cleaning the kitchen and bath, TV time, got them ready for bed, kept them from fighting and kept the doors locked. My children and I had family meetings each day.

When she turned sixteen, I bought her a white day bed with pink comforters, sheets and accessories. This is the one gift I remember getting her because times were financially hard.

I wanted to give her the world! I felt she missed out on being a baby and a child.

She is so much like me with her creative energy as it relates to visualizing tangible things and making them. One time, we partnered up and created crystal jewelry. This was during the 80's before crystal jewelry became so popular. We had a system. Sometimes she'd make sets and I would add the finishings, and there would be times I'd make the sets and she'd add the finishings. We were working in perfect harmony and made lots of money. It was our passion! We worked on this sitting together and drinking coffee, like two old ladies. We shared that happiness together and it will always be there. I think in my heart, I pray in my heart it will overshadow all the pain she was born into, but the reality is, I know that it doesn't. I remember having a reoccurring dream of the two of us walking through Westside Park, in Newark. In the dream, she was about five years. God, I wish my baby's life would have been better!

My baby in pink was born in Martland Medical Center, Newark, NJ.

"Don't worry 'bout a thing, every lil thing's gonna be alright."

Counselor

What would you like to say to your baby in Pink?

Rose

My baby in Pink, please forgive me for introducing you into a world that I allowed to fail you. I am so sorry I didn't give you enough time to snuggle as my baby, nestled in my bosom.

Ma'Me is so heartbroken that you had to receive a heart break before you even knew you had a heart to break.

It pains me that I did not shelter you from outside danger whether it was verbal to you, verbal to someone you love, something you saw, something you had to do, something you did not want to do, something you wanted to do but didn't get a chance to do.

People always say, "the child didn't ask to be here," I say yes, they did ask to be here!

Heaven knew!

This may sound out of the box to some, but I believe that had I not given birth to you, my beautiful baby girl, I would have been blind to the beauty in me. I would not have recognized the Pink in me. Your beauty is my constant affirmation that my life is worthwhile. Your divine presence has been a constant reminder that life is really beautiful. You have shared your beauty by creating beauty in everyone you touch. When I look into a mirror, I see a pretty me because I see you.

I know that your path has been filled with people, places, things, situations, ups, downs and every conceivable bridge over turbulent waters, but I want you to know that I love you so.

You asked to be here. You asked to be born. You had to leave heaven so that I could see myself when I look at you. You have saved my life! I pray that you turn the mirror back on yourself and look deep into where you came from and why you came. I pray you care for yourself and never let you go. Thank you, my beautiful gift from heaven, wrapped in the color Pink.

My second daughter was born in 1975. I knew in my heart she would be my child of courage and determination. April 1974, while living in Rochester, NY, she was conceived.

Two months later, I left Rochester to move to Florida, due to domestic violence. I was two months pregnant with her at the time.

I made the mistake of contacting my other two children's father, the abuser. He relocated to Rochester under the pretense of being a changed man and wanting to be with his family. I fell for it and paid the price of getting beat every day.

Off to the Amtrak train station I ran with three babies and one in my womb. They were three years and under. My two older children, aged two and three, held hands. My third child, Sebek, age four months was held in my left arm and my right hand carried my Morse sewing machine.

My sewing machine had become a means to earn a few dollars. I'd make MGT uniforms and make FOI Fez head crowns and alterations.

The sewing machine was made of metal and was extremely heavy. My stress level was high. I'd been beaten the night before and struggling with three young children and a heavy metal sewing machine was the perfect combination for a miscarriage. My baby held on tight and we went for the ride of our lives, fighting every step of the way. I felt her courage and determination seeping through every part of my body. My need to survive exceeded my own expectations. All I knew was that my baby inside my womb made a difference. I had never felt the energy of fight before. It was present and was determined to stay.

The baby that resided inside my womb, held on! She came to be my Baby in Red. She was the monitor that checked my heartbeat. She asked to be here. Her presence from heaven came in the form of Red.

It is so ironic, once I finally left Hassain and went to Jasper, FL, I ended up contacting him again. I lost confidence in myself and became fearful to do it alone. He came to Jasper when I was eight months pregnant. I was living in a low-income community paying two dollars a month for rent. My grandparents made sure I had furniture and food. My three children were being cared for and I was maintaining my life with all the basic needs including a house phone and color TV. With all the material things I needed and my grandparents being nearby, I still felt empty, alone and could not envision a future. I was blind and worn out from life. I ended up calling him and he convinced me, once again, that he needed to be with his family. At seven months pregnant, I called him and told him to come. I think deep down he really wanted to do the right thing, but both of us grew up in the same neighborhood and neither one of us knew how to change our behavior.

So, once he arrived, he proceeded to beat me over and over again for tricking him into coming to such a small depressing town. He did not help me with the children. He took his frustrations out on me by beating me. In my mind, I needed to do something, but I was more trapped than ever before. I did not have any friends or extra money and there was no bus transportation. This was a small town with one traffic light, supermarket and one hospital.

I had never had a doctor's checkup during my entire pregnancy. When it was time for me to go to the hospital, my grandparents took me. He stayed home and watched the other children. When I arrived, I was in full labor. The birthing experience was extremely frightening and lonely. The nurses literally strapped me at the ankles and wrists. They told me they couldn't risk me injuring myself or creating a problem to the delivery. I was scared shitless. I tried to make eye contact with the big heavy set African American nurse. I wanted her to like me so she would not let harm come to me. I wanted my mother so bad. I had to beg and plead with her in a calm manner under extreme pain to please, please let my wrists free. She eventually let one of them free. I clung onto her hand. It took a long time for my baby to come. I was tense and my body was not in harmony with delivery. I refused to let them inject any pain medication into my body. I didn't trust them. I had to conjure every ounce of courage I had in me in order to let go of the fear that had a hold of me. I knew that I had to be strong. I tried to relax long enough, and I fought like hell to stay awake. I was filled with fear and in an instant, the fear seemed to dissipate, and my baby came.

She is my spirit child. I have spirit because for the first time in my life, I felt her spirit working through me.

She is the child that kept up with me as it relates to physical endurance. She has always spoke with confidence, without hesitation or fear. Her mark is that of a leader.

Growing up, I didn't have a choice but to let her lead. Her competitive spirit showed up on the playgrounds when she competed in races with other children and won. She'd rush home and show me her winning medal or ribbon. I remember when she wanted to get a job. I knew that once she put her mind to something, she wouldn't let it go until she became successful. I also knew that once she started making her own money, it would mark a drastic change in her life. She would acquire an independent behavior that was waiting to go. I was afraid she would want to leave home and get her own apartment. She matured quickly.

I told her she could get a job at age sixteen. I figured sixteen was a safe age, because it would be two years before she was legally old enough to declare her independence. This didn't frighten me, I just had to make the mental adjustment. At age sixteen, she got her first job at the neighborhood library on South Munn Avenue. The staff loved her! She was always articulate, polite and went after a task with great focus and accuracy.

She assisted me when we had a drama ensemble of about sixteen children between the ages of six and thirteen. She was about twelve at the time. She organized, directed and made sure the children had their parts in the plays we performed. Her ability to set a spark to others has also been a strong point in her personality.

There was an extended period in my life when money was extremely scarce. Welfare didn't cut it and any part-time night job helped, but not enough. She worked, as did some of my other children, and helped with paying bills. Her McDonalds job was a blessing because I knew there would be added income in the family. The work ethic of my Child in Red became increasingly relentless as she grew older. I recall her bagging groceries, baby sitting and working for a major corporation. This corporation was name Bellcorp. Only a few select high school students were put at the front of the line for this prestigious job, and she was one of them.

Red's goals and ambition pushed away any ideas of defeat.

Her spirit took on hard outside family tasks, in contrast with my first-born daughter who had more responsibilities indoors. Throughout her high school years, she would take my seventh born child Heru, to Heritage Day Care Center each morning before she went to school.

She'd get on the bus with him, drop him off and catch another bus to her school, Newark Tech. I gave her the freedom to bring her boyfriends to our apartment. I figured with a spirit like hers, if I didn't, she'd find a way to see them. I thought, I'd rather have them visit in her space rather than she go to their space.

When our phone bill needed to get an extension due to nonpayment, she'd call Bell telephone company and negotiate an extension.

She is that child that welcomed a healthy debate. Due to her take charge attitude, she became the captain of the debate team while in high school.

Honor Roll student, in the band playing a flute were part of her goal list.

It was not until later in our lives that we began to clash. It was inevitable. Our fires began to get out of control. Our mother-daughter relationship could have taken a turn for the worst, but we were always determined to figure out how to have a healthy relationship. Our courage and determination reflected each other. We cried, fought and battled with each other. It is our unconditional love that keep us linked. We had to learn this, and it is still a daily endeavor. Through her, I have learned courage, determination and how to control my fire. What a blessing. As a team, we are learning how to balance our energy and not allow it to destroy us. She is my spiritual child. Her heavenly gift presents itself as courage.

 Like a wildfire in a dry forest, we are learning how to control our flames. Our flames, if unattended, will destroy. She is my Red, kick ass spiritual child.

Again, I think that babies ask to be here. Only, they are not babies as we know babies. They are angels in heaven waiting for their call. They are angels waiting in Heaven to come teach us an ultimate lesson about ourselves and in the process, we learn how to raise them, but in fact we are learning how to raise ourselves. As they age, they gain earthly insight which helps them to evolve to the next level of their mundane life. The cycle repeats itself with them having children or them remaining in your life as a permanent guardian angel. The battles come, then the victories if there can be a compromise. However, every step is growth and the Heavens do not discriminate. This is what I believe. My Baby in Red taught me courage. She taught me how to tap into the courage I already had in myself but was covered with fear. She is the spark that keeps me moving and hitting my target. I am thankful to Heaven. *Thank you, Baby in Red, for choosing me as your mother.*

My Baby in Red was born in Hamilton County Hospital, Jasper, Florida.

"Best Friend"

While three months pregnant with my sixth child, daughter number three, my husband, the love of my life, got locked up and would spend the next three years in prison. My entire spirit and world collapsed. Heaven started working on an Angel long before he went to prison. As a matter of fact, the Angel I was carrying decided she needed to arrive ahead of schedule, because I was a mental wreck. I sank into a world of depression.

Marijuana became my husband's replacement. I was convinced it was okay to smoke and besides, the state of mind I was in at the time, it really didn't matter. Morning, noon and night. If my life depended on me telling you how I took care of my other children, I would be dead! My mind and spirit had left my body, yet somehow the hand of a Higher Source pushed, pulled, tugged and guided my blind self along the way. I was done! I did not want to live, but I do not recall wanting to commit suicide. I'm thinking that, if a person gets to the point of wanting to commit suicide, they would not be thinking clearly, anyway. So, I guess I wouldn't remember.

My family were my friends who lived in the Towers. They are my brothers and sisters in spirit who were by my side. I don't remember them being there, but I am certain they were.

Sakyna, she was my number one sister. She is the sister who took me and my four children in from that domestically violent relationship. Our bond was solid. She introduced me to marijuana. We would smoke all night while the children slept. I remember smoking so much one night, I thought I was losing my mind. I believe the shit was so potent and I took too much in. After all, I was a rookie. She talked me back to sanity, because I just knew I was going crazy. I actually remember that night. Sakyna was also a victim of domestic violence. She survived abuse from her grandmother and her husband. The stories she told me were heart wrenching. We'd sit up all night talking and smoking. She was an excellent cook. She'd bake whole wheat bread, fry whiting fish and make zucchini. Those are the three dishes I remember most. And, oh, she'd bake carrot cakes. That sister was the best cook!!!

Sakyna committed suicide from a gun shot in the stomach.

Rock, my spiritual brother, protected and provided for us. He was the brother and still is the brother that I prayed for. I remember one day there was a threat of harm to one of my children. Rock sent a posse of brothers to handle the situation. The dude (grown dude) who was trying to touch my daughter inappropriately, left the state. Rock didn't play when it came to his family. His children were my children and my children were his children. I could not have survived without him!

He is my brother that never said no when the children and I needed something. He had his own family. Hameenah, his children's mother, had the same number of children as I. She was a genius. I always say to myself, she died of a broken heart. Rock loved her and she truly loved him, but she loved drugs more. I'll never forget the heart to heart she and I had one day. It was one of the rare times I saw her not high. She told me she didn't know how to recover from a broken heart. She also said that she loved her family more than anything else. In her mind, if she couldn't make it with Rock, she didn't want to make it.

Years later, she overdosed on heroin.

Jamillah, a younger sister of five years, became so close to me as well. I met her before I moved in with Sakyna. She and her family stood like a barrier between my abuser and me. They lived in the house next to where my four children and I were staying when we got back to Jersey from Jasper. Goldsmith Avenue was beautiful. Jamillah's entire family were God sent. Her mother came to my door one morning, angry, hands on hips and said, "My mother taught me that a man is not supposed to put his hands on a woman." This may sound crazy, but she was the first grown woman to tell me that. It was like, folks knew that I was getting my ass kicked, but not a single soul came to my rescue. I had to learn how to know what I needed to do in order to stay alive. Her words pierced my heart and took the form of courage and fight.

That same night, he came back around. I was petrified when he knocked on the door. Fear will make you do unheard of things. I opened the door. All I remember is him raping me while the children were in the next room sleeping.

In about four weeks, I knew I was pregnant because I missed my period. My body felt pregnant. Any time I'd gotten pregnant, sleepiness would take over.

Week five, I found myself at Beth Israel hospital. They confirmed I was pregnant. The doctor asked what I wanted to do. I told him I did not want to keep the pregnancy. An abortion was scheduled. Jamillah worked as a volunteer at the hospital during that time. I did not know this, so when I saw her there the day of the scheduled abortion, I was surprised. She was a guardian angel during the process before and after. Our friendship grew beyond sisterhood. I do not know where she is to date.

I never had any regrets about the abortion. Afterwards, I tried to put a hit out on him. I contacted some people in Jersey City. I saved my welfare money and had it all lined up for his execution. The people who were supposed to carry it out, reneged. In a way, I'm glad; the authorities probably would have come to my door first.

So, moving to the Weequahic Towers became my first real home with a real circle of love. That is where I met Ab, my children's father. I'll say it again, he was the love of my life and in many unthought of ways, he still is.

Anyway, we had our first child together in 1977. When he got locked up, I was age twenty-two and pregnant. In my care were five children ages ranging from 0 years to 6. I suddenly, without warning, had the love of my life ripped away from me.

It also devastated the children.

I was in grave trouble.

My Angel of Peace is my Baby in Yellow. My pocket full of sunshine, only I didn't know it yet, decided she would come two months early. I believe she knew I was killing myself. Without warning, I went into hard labor. The security guard called the hospital and within a few minutes, the ambulance whisked me away.

My Angel weighed 5 pounds at birth. She came to the world smiling. Her big personality lit up the entire room. I waited for her to cry, but she never did. She was so tiny! I watched her closely; as if I would lose her in the blanket. She didn't have any health problems, so we were able to go home in three days.

On the third day of being in the hospital, my friend Jamillah came to get us. We took a cab back to my apartment. Upon arrival, my five other children greeted us with love and hugs. My son next to her in age was a baby of eleven months.

During those days, the sisterhood was tight. One of the sisters watched all five of the children while I was in the hospital. Without them, I would have been totally lost and alone.

I remember holding my little Angel so gently into my bosom. I was extra careful not to press her too tight. She was the smallest baby I had given birth to. Her ankles were the width of my finger. I still have her hospital bracelet. I was thankful that she didn't have any health problems and that her weight was not too low. The 5-pound mark was safe.

My tiny Angel Baby sparkled like a ray of sun. As I held and watched her, I experienced an energy that I could not explain. It was like she chose me so that I could learn the magic of peace and stillness within. When I looked at her, I could see into her eyes a stillness and calm that I needed. This little Angel knew this. This is why she chose me for her mother. I was in desperate need of calm and peace. I was depressed and sad all the time. Being in the presence of my little Angel, sadness disappeared.

My little Angel cast a spell on me. I'd find myself sitting, staring at her. She was so tiny, I felt I needed to protect and watch over her. I became a little alarmed at the fact I had not heard her cry. I was deeply sad and depressed. My depression was dealt with by me smoking. I never smoked around my Angel and I had almost completely stopped. I didn't know how to live without smoking a joint. I didn't think about the consequences. In the process of me trying to stay alive and alert to care for my other children, I kept my eyes on my quiet and peaceful little Angel. She never cried! Each time I would look over to check on her, it was as if a ray of sunlight came from her tiny body. Such a calm expression on her tiny face. Her gaze looked like she was always playing with the angels. I was compelled to stay close by.

On day six of her life, I glanced over at her as she lay in the center of my bed and she was turning blue!!! I yelled to one of the children to get Sakyna while I hysterically called the security guard downstairs in the lobby and asked him to call an ambulance. The ambulance arrived and took us through the emergency room entrance at Martland Medical Center. My body became numb and it felt as if I was being controlled by a remote controller.

After a million test and tubes hanging from her tiny body, the doctor told me she had literally stopped breathing. It came to be known as SIDS, sudden infant death syndrome. However, she did not die. She stayed in the hospital for six days. My sister-friends took turns watching the other children while I stayed with her.

So, that is who she is, an angel from God! She was sent to wake my ass up to reality. Her presence showed me life and death within the same moment. This Angel has also showed me peace. She inspired the life back into me with her gentle ray of yellow light. Her tiny body withstood the trauma of living inside of my traumatized body for seven months. She came to the world calm and peaceful. She was so calm until she stopped breathing. This Angel came into my life with laughter, smiles, hugs and an angelic voice. I kept her by my side. Her tiny angel wings spread across my broken wings and hovered over them to keep me from falling. I began to rise above my own misery. A spiritual transformation was taking place. Her miracle of birth and living was my miracle of life.

Her life essence expressed warm yellow rays of the sun. She is not a friend of evil, deceit, anger, revenge or any negative emotion that tarnishes the spirit. To this day, she still plays inside with her angel friends; just as she did when she was a baby. She is magical, friendly and we are more than just mother and daughter. We are like two angels playing in the sun, remaining peaceful and calm.

When she was a teenager, I became pregnant with my eighth child. I was so damn tired. I could have laid down in the street and slept through noise and all worldly events. When I finally had my eighth child, she rescued me by helping me take care of her. I was thankful to have the help and love. Her heart has never showed any negative emotion that parents sometimes hear from their children about them doing too much for a sibling. Both of us raised my eighth-born child. They are still attached by the hip.

During high school, she played the saxophone. She looked so pretty in her band outfit. She had skills and played as if it was so natural. Maybe one day she'll play again.

It's so amazing how she has evolved into a full-grown Angel. She plays with them still to this day. As a matter of fact, she collects them, and her home is a scene from Heaven. She included a room for me to come when I need a little calm. She knew then and she knows now.

When she turned eighteen and left home, I had a meltdown that lasted for months. God knew that my wings had healed enough and that I could fly. I simply needed to find calm and peace. I knew I had it.

She is the child that came and turned my life around. I was able to think clearly and make better choices about my future. One major change was to attend college. I could not bear the thought or sight of my six babies and myself sleeping on mattresses on a basement floor. We did this for six months in a cold drab basement on Shanley Avenue, Newark, NJ. It was just my six babies and myself trying to get up out of hell. I thought of how my little Angel looked when she was born and how calm she remained when she went back to the hospital. The thought of her peaceful energy took over my entire body.

I remember as if it were yesterday. She was less than eighteen months. I held her in my arms and said, "Ma'Me needs you to potty, baby. Ma'Me wants to go to college. They won't let me bring you to day care on campus if you are not potty trained." She looked as if she understood what I was saying. Within a day or two of me training her, she never had an accident. She, her brother next to her and I started attending Bloomfield College. This was in 1979.

Thank you, my Angel, for choosing me as your mother. I have watched your wings expand throughout the years. Your calm and peaceful spirit fills my entire body with what has been missing when I am faced with a rational decision. Your yellow essence, which is my inspiration to live, evolved when I witnessed your tiny body lie in a hospital, calm and peaceful in the face of my fear and hysteria. I have learned calm through watching you. I understand peace because you are such a peaceful spirit from Heaven. Thank you for choosing me my beautiful Angel in Yellow.

My Baby in Yellow was born in Martland Medical Center, Newark, NJ.

"Pocket full of Sunshine"

Therapist

Somewhere inside of you there is a strong and courageous woman. She's coming out more each day. Were you still using during this time?

Rose

During and after my sixth child, I was smoking a little. I began using cocaine in 1981. I used throughout my college days and beyond. I stopped using cocaine when I nearly overdosed in 1988. Had it not been for my sister-friend Shirley, I would have. There was a snowstorm outside. We stayed inside talking and using our drug of choice all night into the next morning. My son Heru was about seven months. I remember her holding me up and walking me to the fire escape. As we walked through the house to reach the fire escape, I recall my daughter in Red sitting and holding my baby Heru. She had stomach cramps, yet she still clung on to him as my friend escorted me out to the cold wind in a desperate effort to save my life. She talked to me and kept me from passing out. I remember sinking into a state of darkness. It almost felt good and relieving. I told her to take me to the hospital because I was really scared. She told me if she took me to the hospital, they would take my children due to drug abuse. At that moment, I began to fight. She told me to calm down and to breathe slowly. I did everything she told me to do. I remember the image of my daughter in pain holding on to her brother. She was about thirteen years at the time. I think I used about two or three times afterwards. In between me finally stopping the use of cocaine, I ended up in the emergency room at least once for a fast beating heart. The medical team did not check for drug use. I was thankful for that. It was rough, but the thought of me losing my children outweighed the use of drugs. I stopped cold turkey. It was during this time I began to drink Guinness Stout. I drank a bottle in the morning, afternoon and before bed.

Therapist

Tell me about your fourth daughter.

Rose

I was thirty-seven and pregnant with my eighth child and fourth girl. This meant I would be delivering a baby at thirty-eight. What the hell was the matter with me, was all I could think. It appeared on the surface that my life was going right, so how in the hell did I allow myself to get pregnant again. Another self-imposed 'body punch.' I was ashamed, embarrassed and a touch of angry. When I finally let go of the shame, embarrassment and anger, I prayed for a girl.

Throughout my pregnancy, I faced challenges that tested my faith and my stress level was high. It took all I had in me to continue work. I was embarrassed. I was supposed to be the example, yet here I was pregnant at thirty-seven and without a husband. Confusion cluttered my head and my self-image and esteem suffered. Anxiety was taking over. I was tapped out!

I had been living in the fast lane of life, all my life. I was doing a million things, including getting pregnant.

Therapist

What do you mean, "the fast lane"?

Rose

I was so busy doing so many things without coming up for air. Working, my family, my business, men, art and anything else that served as a distraction from me looking at myself or my mental sloppiness. So many of my sister and brother-friends had fallen into a realm of environmental and situational hopelessness. We were simply going through the motions of life, repeating the same mistakes over and over. We did not realize it. We thought we were making progress. In some instances, we were. However, the same energy in the air that we breathed consumed us and we'd find ourselves always back to square one.

Deep inside, I felt that I had let my family down. Words could not express to them how terrible I felt, nor could I think about it in depth. I tried to keep a little dignity about myself. Holding on to faith faded more with each day. Faith in what? Look forward to what?

The father of my baby showed me a part of himself that sent me over the edge. I wore the face of the so-called strong woman and continued to be the rock for so many, but inside I was wandering in an emotional cesspool. My body continued to function on the outside, but my insides were a mangled pile of other folk's shit.

My pregnancy progressed as I continued to work, doubting myself and feeling numb to reality every step of the way. Thank goodness I didn't crave cocaine; I was always tired.

Walking into the classroom with a baby bump was embarrassing and shameful.

Therapist

Yes, but it took a tremendous amount of courage and faith!

Rose

Thank goodness for courage and faith!

My students knew I wasn't married, and it mattered what they thought of me. Here I was, sporting myself as an example and ended up pregnant with an eighth child and no husband.

I underestimated my students. They did not question me or look at me differently. They were actually happy for me, embraced me with love and so did the staff. One thing that folks who don't understand about the culture in the 'hood' is that we experience the same type of environmental shit. What might look like dysfunction to one group, is perfectly normal in another group.

Depression, desperation, abuse and sadness often became a way of life. In our environment, self-medication was the way so many of us dealt with the never talked about problems and issues we were born into and experienced. Seeking out a counselor or therapist was not in our vocabulary. Our secrets about what went on in our individual families was ours to hold. We had to appear as if our lives were on the right track. We looked at anyone going to a counselor as being crazy; crazy house crazy!

I didn't know then, but I later discovered that my pregnancy was the Heaven sending me the gift of Chi, breath. My Chi, Baby in Orange, chose me because she knew I had to breathe. But in order to breathe I had to have faith. She came from Heaven as my Baby in Orange.

On January eleventh, I went into labor and birthed a beautiful baby daughter.

Let me back up a bit.

I was still navigating on automatic while hiding extreme exhaustion throughout my pregnancy.

I was hanging onto a thin, short thread that showed frayed and withered fibers. No one was able to see the inside of my withered and tired spirit. All folks saw was what I wanted them to see. My baby was so beautiful and regardless of how long and tiring my day was, her smile brought me joy.

My children were angry that I had gotten pregnant and had another baby. It seemed as though having babies was all I knew how to do. It just so happened I got pregnant about six weeks after her birth. I suffered a miscarriage and nearly died. My body was shutting down. The only one who knew this was her father. I remember us taking the bus to the emergency room. The doctors did what they had to do, including tying my tubes to prevent any future pregnancies.

Taking the bus back home proved to be painful and tiresome. He nearly had to carry me, as I could barely walk. That's all I remember, except I did have a certain feeling that if I got through this episode, I would be able to get through anything. I made a promise to God that I would pray each day to do better and to please, please don't take my children's mother away from them. My daughter in Yellow was taking care of my newborn Baby in Orange while I attended my medical needs in and out of the hospital.

The rest of my children were in the care of my daughter in Pink, my eldest child.

I had created a family mess. Even though my children seemed to still love me, I knew they were unhappy. I didn't know how to get out of this cycle of self-destructive decisions. I always thought I was making good choices until things would get turned upside down.

Therapist

What did you do after you settled in after having the baby?

Rose

In May of 1995, the Friday before Mother's Day, my mother called. She told me that my grandmother asked if I was ok with relocating to Florida to take care of the family home. My grandmother was not doing well. I told my mother I would think about it. My mind and spirit became very relaxed and there weren't any hints of fear and doubt. I really didn't know what the future held but I felt deep within that something great was happening. I kept feeling an unending surge of faith. I didn't want to know what was going to happen. I did know, that with such a move, it had to place my children and I in a better situation. So, without knowing, God knew.

On Mother's Day 1995, I woke up bright and early, called my mother and told her, yes, I would relocate. In three months' time, my three youngest children and I had moved to Jasper, Hamilton County, Florida.

The move literally saved my life and I am certain it also saved my children's lives.

For the first time in my life, I began to see and feel less doubtful. The decision to relocate boosted my self-confidence.

My Baby in Orange was quiet and always had a smile on her face without physically smiling. Her presence and expression slowed my breathing down because I was so tired, I didn't know what else to do. I'd hold her on my chest after nursing and our breath would sync up together. I nursed her a lot. Also, I knew she was the last child I would birth.

We finally moved to Hamilton County. Eventually, I began to see life from a different perspective. I was able to pay attention to this beautiful little girl without having the distractions, confusion and discomforts of yesterday.

Her little hands would always feel and trace the surface of my face as if she was speaking words. My breathing became in sync with her breathing. This little child who restored my breath was actually teaching me how to breathe and not allow stress to enter.

Before we left New Jersey, our favorite getaway was downtown Newark, in front of the PSE&G (Public Service Electric & Gas) building. In front of the building was a big water fountain and mountains of steps that led into the building. We'd go there, sit on the bottom row of steps closest to the water and stay for hours. The sound of the water drowned out all the noise in my head. She was fascinated by the water sounds, as well. We would share a sandwich, water and sometimes apple juice. This was our place of calm. We'd always end up there after leaving the welfare building, aka Social Services, on Broad Street. That place was a jungle that I refuse to visit in my head.

So, there we were, in small town Jasper. I didn't know what to think. I just went with the flow. I was able to look at my two-year-old baby and for the first time in my life as a mother, experience the depth of having a baby. I was actually breathing! There was no stress and worry about being evicted, no food, electric shut off, the hustle and bustle of going to work every day and dealing with the stress of co-workers and students. And not to mention the shame, guilt and embarrassment I felt towards my other children for letting them down and allowing a stranger into our home. I believe my Baby in Orange chose me to teach me how to breathe. She knew that her presence would release me from being in such a shameful, confused and stressful frame of mind. My pregnancy would create a chain of events that would remove me from people, places and things, so that I could learn how to breathe.

While living in Jersey, I never had time to breathe. Hell, I didn't know how to breathe. I went through a lot of automatic motions that lie dormant inside of me, waiting for an opportunity to be released.

I believe the main reason I decided to relocate to Florida was because of my Baby in Orange.

When we got settled into our home, I began to think about what I wanted for my three minor children that were there. My other five children remained in New Jersey. My Herukhuti was eighteen at the time and did not want to relocate. I regret not making a lot of fuss about him not coming. Maybe it's just as well because when he decided to relocate to Florida, it was because he wanted to and not because I convinced him to come.

Anyway, back to my Chi. It occurred to me that my baby liked dancing. So, I found a dance studio and enrolled her. She danced so gracefully! Her movements at age two brought attention to the dance instructor who found it hard to openly acknowledge. The instructor's daughter was also a student and had two left feet. Seeing was believing at the recital. My baby was a winner! Orange continued to dance through-out elementary school. She took ballet and jazz lessons. I didn't force her, she did it naturally. She also played the violin from third through twelfth grade.

I enjoyed going to her concerts! During high school, she was required to dress in a long formal black dress with black heels. She looked so elegant.

Home practice became soothing. She'd practice for hours and after she felt she'd mastered a particular piece, she'd ask me to listen to it. Her playing was steady, calm and strong. I got a kick out of watching her body move with the notes.

We became a team for the performing arts. I'd be in my room, listening to her rehearse on her violin or sit and watch while she rehearsed her dance steps.

She also drew and painted pictures for me almost every day. She wrote and illustrated her first book for me at age three. She'd always end it with "I did it". Her little hands sculpted figurines out of pipe cleaners. Her ability to create allowed me to see how much faith she had in herself to start something and finish it or not finish it. If there was a time that she did not finish a project, she didn't get upset with herself. She'd simply start something else or create a different approach; all while remaining calm.

I recall being so stressed out one day. It was as if my whole life came rolling through my head at once. I had a couple of dollars stacked to the side for a rainy day. She had to be about eight years. At the time, we were living in Tallahassee, Florida. I decided for us to go on a little over night retreat. Once we arrived at a little bed and breakfast, I lie helplessly in bed. However, I awakened to a different me. My little Orange had made my face up using her Disney make-up kit. She also covered my entire body with citrus body cream. At that moment I knew that everything was going to be alright.

Our favorite things to do together were straight out of what some folks call a 'nerds handbook'. For example, we would binge on Storm Stories, The Wild Thornberrys, Survival type programs, go to museums, sit on the beach in our favorite spot, Epcot and things related to the planets and stars. We became vegetarians together, love ourselves some Tropical Smoothie, and our walnut strawberry salads was to live for. I learned how to live a different life. I took note of what I enjoyed, what I wanted to do and the things that made me happy.

We didn't like a lot of company or talking on the phone. Being alone in our world was the best place to be. We would mingle with others from time to time, but we'd always be in our world. We felt good there and did not feel the need to be apologetic about it.

If anyone had the ability to spiritually create an inner awareness for me to stop and smell the flowers, it was my Baby in Orange. I am thankful to know how to breathe because she chose me for her mother. She is my Chi in the midst of storms. I am thankful to be alive.

Thank you, my Baby in Orange, for choosing me as your mother.

I know how to breathe.

My Baby in Orange was born in Beth Israel Hospital, Newark, NJ.

"Don't Stop Til You Get Enough"

Session #15

Bedtime brings laughter

Night dreams appear from the stars

Birth of a new day

Therapist

What is something you are able to look forward to doing each day? Something that you think you will enjoy doing!

Keep it simple. It doesn't need to be something that requires money.

Rose

I've always enjoyed writing. When I was a little girl, I remember writing poems. I'd leave them on top of my mother's dresser. She would always leave me a nickel in the place of my Dick and Jane poems.

So, yeah! I really enjoy writing! Also, I love riding a bike. I rode my friend's bike when I was a child. I think I rode it more than she rode it.

Therapist

Okay! That's great. Get yourself a bike and start riding and writing. That's doable.

DEAR GOD

Rose

I am somewhere, yet nowhere.

My mind, body and spirit are overwhelmed.

Each moment I struggle to keep my inside light shining.

I know that it remains on because of You.

Times when I was sure to die, You illuminated within me even more.

Times when I had nothing, You showed me I had everything.

Dear God, at this time my spirit holds emptiness, my mind is stretched, and my body is listless.

I am still standing, walking, talking and even manage to smile, because of Your grace and mercy.

My mother is doing well, my children and grandchildren are healthy, I am living in a beautiful home, my life is of art, walking on the shoreline is my past time and hunger is not felt.

My dear God, I am having a problem letting go of this constant cloud of hopelessness.

My happy is buried and I do not know how to think or feel long term images of light.

Dear God, I am sad, overwhelmed and crying inside!

Day in and day out I watch her tired, fragile body while listening to all the abuse she has endured throughout her entire life. Her silent tears of pain and hurt is more than I can bear.

I love her so much and I am doing my best for her, which appears to not be enough.

Dear God, my mother has been in pain since age three. One miserable experience after another. A love that was promised to her turned into a never-ending nightmare.

Her stories paint pictures with gory details of her father beating her mother with his fists and dragging her through the house like a rag doll. This is how she remembers her father. She said she loved her father, Dear God!

The stories she tells of him drinking and referring to her as a boy and not his little girl still plagues her mind. Tears are suppressed as stories continue, one after the other of how she tried desperately to protect her mother at the cost of her tiny body being whirled against the wall or knocked to the floor. Her five-year-old strength was no match, yet she'd return and fight some more.

She worked and suffered in the tobacco and cotton fields in the blazing hot sun, Dear God.

She prayed for relief, but it never came. Instead, she ended up in a deeper Hell.

I am her daughter, she is my mother, I am her caregiver. I hear her stories. I see her body. I feel her pain and hurt. It has thrown me off balance to realize that I am unable to erase the hurt and memories of her misery. She is my mother.

Dear God, I am scattered across the floor after being torn into thousands of pieces.

Her stories are plastered in my head and are my everyday thoughts. I do not know what to do.

Stress and anxiety welcome me as tensions rise high.

I am challenged to redirect her thoughts, but quickly defeated.

Anxiety and stress have won again!

Dear God, I just want to get in my bed, pull the covers over my head and go to sleep.

Yet, I am afraid of sleep.

Nightmares of my past awake me to a trembling body drenched in sweat and an exhausted mind.

Dear God

I want to escape!

I cringe while walking on my trip back home.

My heart automatically starts to pound.

I am fifteen, again.

I am paranoid, Dear God!

Each move that I make I feel as though I am being watched.

It better be the right move or I will be scolded or given the silent treatment.

"You're too quiet! Are you sick? I don't like when you don't talk. Why are you in that room so long? I'm not used to people not talking!"

No one is listening!

Dear God

I embrace the silence! It frees me of the constant turmoil inside my head.

I welcome my ability to withdraw from the outside.

People are quick to say what I should feel like and what I should do. They are quick to say

"You should enjoy these moments."

I say to them, "Go to hell! You do not know me, you do not live with me! If you want to do something, HELP ME!"

They also say, "Cherish your mother while she is alive."

I DO CHERISH HER!

What does cherish and feeling unhappy have to do with one another?

I am not feeling happy.

I do not know how to be happy in the midst of unhappiness.

My mother and I cry every day without either one of us knowing.

Dear God

Help me to reignite my light. I am getting cold.

I feel a warm flicker from time to time.

I know the flicker is a manifestation of your Omnipresence.

Help me dear God.

Yes, I still pray.

Dear God

I'm listening really hard, but I can't turn my thoughts off.

Guide me, protect me, help me to let go of the images, thoughts and memories of yesterday.

Help me to take steps toward helping myself. Help me to not drift into tomorrow, only to become overwhelmed with what it may bring.

Help me to stand up straight in this moment and remember happiness.

Sadness is such a welcomed color in my heart.

Help me to become aware of this musty energy that reaches my nose and prevents me from breathing. Help me, Dear God, to pray it away.

Dear God

I am ...

I am living in the world but not of the world.

Trying hard not to drift away in a cloud of colorless emotions.

Dear God

Once upon a time I felt joy in my tears as they streamed down my cheeks to cleanse my spirit.

I am in need of a good cleansing.

I have neglected my responsibility of cleaning and caring for my spirit, Dear God.

If I cry. I may not be able to stop.

I come to you, Dear God.

I'll go to the mountains and form a river.

I went to the mountains and the river never came.

Talking to you out loud worked better.

I was able to turn off my thinking.

Thank you for a real conversation!

I so depend on you.

Now, I randomly speak out to you.

People look at me as if I am crazy.

I don't care if people think that I am crazy.

I am getting better.

Dear God

What shall I do when my way out pushes me deeper in?

I joined a group on social media.

Help for Caregivers of Elderly Parents.

My letter to them; "I am grateful to be a member of the group. I have been really trying to maintain a sense of emotional balance since becoming the caregiver for my mother. She is currently 91. We have been living together since June, 2019. However, she has been in my care since July 11, 2018. I am experiencing a mountain of mixed emotions. I am certain many, if not all of you, can relate. I have connected with this group because I know that isolation with my thoughts about this particular journey of caring for my mother is not healthy. Thank you."

Dear God

Last night, I woke up to a loud bump coming from my mother's room.

Within a split second, I ran to her room. She had fallen off the bed and was now on the floor.

Upon reaching the room, I quickly lifted her body up. In my mind, if I lifted her fast enough, time would reverse, and she wouldn't be on the floor from a fall.

Thank you, Dear God, for placing an Angel beneath her to catch her fall.

At night, I lay awake, while I am asleep.

I am afraid she will fall.

"Just for this moment, Dear God"

SESSION #16

Free bird returns home

Cherry blossom tree is bare

Rain falls from bird's beak

Rose

Today, I cried.

SESSION #17

———

Blue bird of patience

Shivers at the sight of rain

Slept through the spring storm

Therapist

How are you feeling?

Rose

My feelings are persistent and scattered. It's hard for me to breathe.

Therapist

Yes, but how do you feel?

Rose

Although I am surrounded by people who love me, I feel alone. I feel as though my body is not moving in harmony with my mind. Then suddenly, my thoughts begin to race, and my body reacts with heavy breathing.

Therapist

Focus on your thoughts just before the onset of the heavy breathing. What were your thoughts or what were you doing prior to or during the breathing?

Rose

It sometimes happens just before I get up from bed, about to come home from a walk or a simple walk from my bedroom to the kitchen. My mind starts to race without any clear mental explanation that I am able to pinpoint. That's the best I am able to come up with, after giving your question some thought.

Therapist

Something has happened in the past that places you in this fight or flight mode. Your body immediately remembers. In time, you will be able to think about and learn the triggers that set you into that uncomfortable mode. Tell me, during that particular moment, how do you recover?

Rose

I just try to breathe. I look at my Fitbit to see what my BPM is. I try to avoid moments when I know I will experience anxiety.

I stay out for long periods of time. And there are other times, I get up before the sun rise so I can leave the house. I tiptoe around and keep the lights off so as not to be heard.

Therapist

Why do you need to stay out for long periods, leave the house so early, tiptoe and keep the lights off?

Rose

Because it's hard to be in my mother's presence. I anticipate a painful conversation before it happens. I know that the conversation will end up like it has always ended up; with pain, hurt or some tragedy. We can be laughing and talking about a good memory. Then out of nowhere a tragedy or abuse story is injected. I have tried over and over to redirect the conversation, but it doesn't work. So, I walk away or sit and become numb. With every conversation.

Unhappiness and hopelessness creeps in and follows me throughout the day.

Therapist

Do you think she will talk to a therapist?

Rose

No, she will never talk to a counselor! She is from the old, old school.

Therapist

What brings you relief?

Rose

Walking! When I am out walking, I am fine. I am totally removed from the situation. As long as I don't think about going home, I am fine. I enjoy being alone in my silence, if that makes sense. It's not that I don't want to have a conversation with my mother, but every conversation turns into an abusive horror story about her father, my father or two of her past husbands. I know my mother has post-traumatic stress. She's in her 90's. I know she is finally living her best life. She needs to be happy and healthy. I realize that her life is tied into her painful past. She shares it all the time and does not think it is causing a problem. If she found out it was hurting me to the extent that it is, it would deeply sadden her and cause her to be in a state of perpetual unhappiness.

I am not sure what to do. This is her story and it is also my story. While she tells her story, I am reliving her story as well as my story. I love her and understand, but this is a double-edged sword that is slicing me into a million pieces.

I will always take care of her, but I don't have a handle on taking care of myself. I am simply going through the motions.

Therapist

What are your thoughts during that time, do you recall?

Rose

My thoughts are…. What are my thoughts? I don't recall any thoughts.

I get filled up with emotions.

My spirit feels emotionally trapped within a continuous flow of unhappy and unconscious feelings. It occurs over and over throughout the day without my permission.

There is no forward movement with my life. Most folks looking in from the outside would probably say differently. On the surface, they see a happy well-grounded woman.

Well, this woman has been carrying a secret for too long.

Did I tell you that my heart flutters to see my mother drag around the house in pain and to hear her moan out loud of her aches and to literally sing songs of dying?

By the way, I woke up at 3am Wednesday morning. I experienced a rush of heart beats as I searched to find my peace. With the nightlight shining, I was able to see into the closet that's connected to my bedroom. I see shadows of dirty clothes spilling over the laundry basket, a crate of shoes piled high and a cramped assortment of unorganized dresses, blouses and jeans hanging from the long rod that reached from one end of the closet to the other.

I guess it's time for me to clean out my closet!

I struggle to keep the scattered puzzle pieces from getting lost before I have a chance to put the puzzle together.

Session #18

Green bird flying high

Wingspan covers the ocean

Free and peace in sky

Therapist

Tell me what you mean when you say you feel hopeless.

Rose

When I am feeling hopeless, I want to stay inside myself. I do not want to be seen and I do not want to talk. It's dark inside and I am not able to find my way out. For some reason, I'm ok with being inside because there is nothing outside. I want to be left alone and not be around anyone. I feel depleted of life, tired and my body and my mind is disconnected. If I am with someone, I am still inside and alone. I am on automatic from how I remember myself to be.

Therapist

What are some instances that cause you to become emotional?

Rose

I am not sure what the exact causes are. It is not just one thing. It can be something small. I really don't describe myself as emotional. I may get stressed or anxiety might creep in. Sometimes, in order to control the situation, I must shut down and not talk. Sometimes I get angry. It really depends on what the situation is.

When someone tries to change me and make me into what they think I should be, I get angry. Or, if someone tries to control me, I get angry. On the other hand, I'm happy when I play and laugh with my grandson at the beach, go out for pizza or have a picnic. I'm also happy when I'm riding my bike. My feelings are hurt when I'm not accepted for who I am. Right now, I'm feeling alone, lost and hopeless.

Therapist

Do you believe that your feelings of hopelessness will change?

Rose

I'm not sure how to change it.

Therapist

Start with telling yourself you are not hopeless. Plant a picture of what you see as being the opposite of hopelessness.

This is where a seed of subconscious hopefulness is planted. You may not feel or believe it at this point, but it is important that you flip your thought process around. And yes, you will get some interference with fear and doubt. That's normal. When it happens, take a deep breath.

We are at the point in our conversations where you will start to do certain things that will increase your ability to cope with moment to moment situations.

This path will be a gradual lifestyle change that allows you to consciously focus on healing your body, mind and spirit. Eventually, your subconscious will take over. The changes will create a complete awareness of who you are and the beauty of why you are the woman you have become. The change will also catch and nip in the bud any potential adverse actions that may come as a result of your emotions. Your emotions and feelings are a part of who you are. They can be sad, happy, resentful, joyous, create anger, excitement or hopelessness. However, they will always be a part of you. You will discover realistic and practical ways in which to cope with them. In doing so, they will lose the power to hurl you into a world of depression, anxiety or post-trauma. Your strength for change lies within.

Rose

So, are you saying, I'm going to be okay?

Therapist

Yes! You will be okay, if you believe you'll be okay.

Do *you* believe you'll be okay?

Rose

Yes, I believe I'll be okay!

Therapist

Great!

We will veer to the next path of your life, one step at a time.

Welcome to your *Healing Path.*

Your life will spiral upward, and you will learn to relax and breathe along the way. You will ventually enjoy and look forward to life.

Rose

Looking forward to life; I'm looking forward to that!

Therapist

The moment you made the decision to seek out a therapist and actually carry through with getting the help you knew you needed, was the moment your life changed.

I will simply lay down the blueprint, but you will do what is necessary for change.

Here we go!

PART THREE
Healing Path

Session #19

Therapist

Let's start with a prayer. Your prayer is your direct line of communication to a Higher Power, your Higher Power. You do not need to be religious to believe in a Higher Power.

Rose, what is your prayer?

Rose

I pray for peace and love for myself, family and the world!

I pray to love myself as I am.

I pray to understand and accept where I have been, where I am.

I pray to call on faith as I move forward with peace and love for myself, my family and the world.

Therapist

Okay, now close your eyes and pray it from the heart.

Rose

My Prayer

Dear God, I am your child and you know me better than I know myself.

Please wrap your arms of peace and love around my body. Allow me to feel your warmth with each breath that I take.

Bless my family and show them mercy.

Help the people in the world to stop hurting each other with hateful words and actions.

Dear God, help me to take better care of myself. Help me to not neglect myself and to remember that I am important for me to love.

Dear God, help me to stop making excuses for myself about things I am able to do.

Dear God, forgive me.

Therapist

Forgiveness. It is a powerful healing prayer.

Rose

Yes, I know and yes, I need forgiveness. I need my children to forgive me.

Therapist

What are you asking them to forgive you for?

Rose

I am asking my children to forgive me for…. okay, here is what I will say to them;

My beautiful, precious children, forgive me for being so caught up in my life's shit that it blinded me to the pain and hurt I was putting you through and all the other horrible shit you experienced and endured due to my ignorance.

Forgive me for not being there for you and being aware of the fact that *m*fer's could have been hurting, abusing and destroying your beautiful spirit.*

Forgive me for not hugging you enough, for not telling you I love you enough, for not holding you into my arms and looking deep into your eyes and picking up on the fact that something could have been wrong.

Forgive me, my beautiful babies, my children, my flesh and blood for ever hurting you with words and for not nursing you in my bosom long enough.

Forgive me for not allowing you to be babies and creating situations that caused you to grow up too soon.

Forgive me, my children, for breaking your heart.

Therapist

Is there someone you would like to forgive?

Rose

Not yet.

Therapist

Let's talk about an affirmation for a moment.

An affirmation is a positive mental and/or visual message. The activation of this message coordinates our breathing by releasing adverse emotions and breathing in the positive energy from the affirmation. It is a reminder that we are exactly who we say we are.

It is an inspirational and motivational message. It affirms your light.

Let's think about our breath for a moment. We know there is an in and out cycle to breathing.

For this conversation, we will call this breath cycle, Yin and Yang.

Yang is in, Yin is out. Yang is the positive, Yin is the negative.

For example, we breathe in courage, we breathe out fear. Don't see it as good or bad. Think in terms that both energies are present. We determine how and when to use the energy and whether we need to invoke it or not.

Courage can be useful at times, but other times it may need to take a step to the side. Think about this. You will not let your courage lead you into acting out a deadly dare, would you? Or, in a split second, the role of fear could save your live. We need both and we have both. We have the ability to decide when we use them. If we have an imbalance and need a dose of courage, we can create an affirmation to stimulate our breathing with a message created to awaken the courage within.

Sometimes we get stuck in Yin.

Place your hands on top of each other in the center of your chest. Close your eyes for a moment. Imagine you are in a river of darkness (Yin) trying to swim across to the river of light (Yang).

Keep in mind the rivers only appear to be separate, but they are one in the same.

Now imagine that you are struggling so hard to get to the light but the more you struggle, the longer you remain where you are.

Now, take a deep breath in (light) and as you breathe out (dark) allow your body to relax.

At the same time you are breathing in, imagine yourself merging with the river of light. Although you are still connected with the river of darkness, you realize that it is a part of you but not harming you. With this awareness and your coordinated breathing, your body becomes relaxed. Now, replace the dark and light with rivers of fear and courage. Breathe in courage, breathe out fear. Feel your body relax. Both exist, but you have control with your breathing.

What do you feel?

Rose

I feel my body relaxing. My breathing has slowed down.

Therapist

Yes. You are allowing the emotion of fear to take its course by breathing it out. Breathing in courage is reviving. Once the coordination of the breath is complete and practiced, you become more aware of your true abilities and inner strength.

Rose

Struggling depletes me and creates anxiety. I don't make progress. It just seems like I'm going nowhere. So, breathing helps me to relax.

Where does the affirmation come in?

Therapist

Right! I'll reiterate. Yin and Yang are equally important. Our goal is to let the process of energy take its course, but we are the navigators. We decide how long and which direction we go or the need to go. Embracing who we are, and breathing is fundamental.

Our emotions are a part of us. We should never struggle with our emotions. Instead we should release them.

The more we learn to accept and understand them, we become self-aware and empowered.

Part of our journey is to evolve and become aware of why and how we have become who we are and improve each day to get better. Our knowledge of this helps us to understand and accept others. It becomes a conscious choice as to whether we want to keep certain energy around us.

Your affirmation should be a simple positive Yang statement, phrase, word or image that you feel and believe. It has to be from you, not from me or anyone else. It should be a verbal expression, image or a combination of both, created to move you forward with love and light and not suppress or stunt your breathing.

It also serves as an expression that will distract you from an unwanted thought so that your energies are able to be redirected.

Rose

Yeah, I know how those unwanted thoughts are, they lead me to negative actions.

Therapist

Exactly! Something that will instantly clear your thought pattern and relax your body with a few breaths.

Session #20

Rose

I am a cool breeze of fresh air on a hot summer's day!

Therapist

I can actually see and feel it! It's definitely you. I like how you associated yourself with nature!

Rose

Oh, yeah! I'll close my eyes and feel the cool breeze flow throughout my entire body to cool me off and calm me down.

Rose

What's your affirmation?

Therapist

My current affirmation is more of a visual. I am standing on a white sand shoreline, facing the ocean, listening and watching blue waves roll in.

Rose

I think I'll need to use that one from time to time!

Therapist

That's fine!

Let's talk about breathing in color.

Rose

That sounds interesting! Tell me about it.

Therapist

It's about the energy we already have and how to use it to achieve optimal mental, physical and spiritual health and wellness. It puts the WHOLE into *Wholistic*.

Color is a living burst of energy that resonates inside of us, around us and within nature.

It is our inner and outer world. It's color that keeps us alive. It is the breath we take in, the foods we eat, nature, the clothes we wear, the color schemes for our homes and the list is endless.

We are not always conscious of it, but we naturally gravitate to certain things in nature and certain colors more than other things.

Our bodies, minds and spirits are subconsciously breathing in and healing from color and nature.

Remember all those long walks on the beach, staring at the turquoise water, cloud gazing, walks through the park, breathing and smelling flowers? You go to a boutique on a spring morning in search of a light blue outfit and you just had to get a red automobile? This is how color reveals itself to you based on what is going on inside from a spiritual perspective. Also, there are certain foods in nature you enjoy more than others. They are sort of like your, 'go to' foods. This is your body letting you know there is a physical need. It is also based on nature's colors. I am not talking about the flesh from animals of creatures from the ocean.

The energy from color breathing is *Wholistic*. It heals our mind, body and spirit.

We will be approaching the application or practice of color breathing from a spiritual perspective.

Your favorite color probably dominates your wardrobe.

Also, there are certain colors you probably won't wear because you do not like them.

When it comes to nature and color, *all* the choices are healing and revealing.

The reds, oranges, yellows, greens, light and dark blues and purples.

The sun, water, earth and air are equally important and necessary in preventing, maintaining and healing our *Whole Selves*.

Prayer, affirmations, color choices, deep breathing, color meditation, meditation and nature are our spiritual resources that will prevent, maintain and heal our Whole Selves.

Rose

Will my affirmation ever change? And how do I meditate with color?

Therapist

Yes! And so will your prayer. I will teach you how to meditate. Nature will kick in. You will naturally gravitate to certain colors, foods and outdoor activities will increase or change.

Rose

I understand a little more about color. I suppose that's why I like certain colors during certain times. There is always something about the summer that pushes me to get a new red dress. And when I think about it, I can never go to sleep with black night clothes on.

I know my mind and spirit will get better, but what about my body?

I'm not sure I understand the connection.

Therapist

Your food intake will gradually change for the better. Not because of a restriction or you denying yourself of certain foods due to a vegetarian diet or some other popular diet, but because of the way you begin to *feel* and *think* about yourself, as a *Whole*.

You'll start to think a lot more about color. The vibrant colors will resonate with your spirit. This will include how you select beautifully colored foods that are from nature.

Your spirit knows what it needs. Sometimes our minds are so conditioned to want what we want, habits are formed, and fast foods and lifeless, colorless foods take over.

Your cravings will change, and awareness of life and living will evolve to a higher level of understanding. For instance, eating a red apple and a plate of green salad will be different. Your knowledge of color and the breathing in of the color subconsciously, will benefit your body, mind and spirit. Balance is the key.

When you go into the grocery store to purchase food, you will start to naturally lean towards nature's colorful foods.

Your choices in snacks will change and meals will become more balanced.

Your energy level will change. You might start walking more, dancing around to music heard only in your head and that bike you told me that is taking up space in your bedroom, may get some use. Rose, you will start to feel better, which will keep the wheels of doing better moving and ultimately you will get better.

Your healing path is *Wholistic*. That means, your mind, body and spirit will be healed simultaneously. It appears to be separate, but it is not.

When you speak your affirmation, you are giving yourself permission to restart. Your mind is rebooted, which unconsciously directs your body to stabilize self and your breathing allows peace to surface so that your spirit will heal.

Rose

You make it sound so relaxing and easy. I am willing to try whatever I need to do, to feel better. I am tired of carrying around feelings of sadness and hopelessness. I feel in my heart, for the first time in my life, someone is not only listening, but are offering realistic ways to get better and feel better. And I don't need to run out a buy a bunch of stuff that ends up taking up space in my home.

Therapist

So good to hear your level of enthusiasm, Rose.

Let me talk about the SWEA for a moment. SWEA is an acronym for: Sun, Water, Earth and Air.

We are a combination of the *sun, water, earth and air.* This combination is vital for our existence.

Lots of sun for energy, water for moisture, earth for food and air to breathe. Take away any one of these natural healers, and we suffer from dis-ease. Too little of any of these natural healers and we suffer from dis-ease. The sun, water, earth and air in its most natural and purest form is what we need for optimal health and wellbeing.

Personally, I love and understand the SWEA so much that I have adopted the SWEA into my life to signal an acknowledgement of the type of meditation I teach.

The logo is a yellow tree with seven roots. The tree is a symbol representing that we are rooted or connected to the sun, water, earth and air and the seven roots connects us to one another.

How we evolve into compassionate, loving and peaceful human beings is determined by how well we care for our *Whole Selves*. In another way of putting it, we have a life task of keeping weeds and bushes from growing and getting between our roots. Those weeds and bushes are negative humans whom we are connected to, unhealthy food, not enough water, and forgetting how to breathe. Our energy becomes depleted because the source of our energy is covered with dark clouds of thought. You've heard the term, "Nip it in the Bud." Well, that means when unhealthy or unwanted stuff starts to develop, we need to pull all those weeds and bushes that hinders our growth, from the roots.

Rose

That makes sense.

So, you said my prayer and affirmation will change, right?

Therapist

Yes! You'll sense when it happens; embrace it.

You will always be in constant motion. Your breathing is your motion. It's a good thing to be in motion. The opposite is death.

Your thoughts, feelings and actions are constantly changing based on how you breathe.

What you will have working in your favor will be awareness.

Once your awareness strengthens, your subconscious will take over at times, and your conscious will inject itself with positive thoughts at other times.

You'll also be able to note the changes your body makes when certain thoughts start to develop.

For instance, is your heart pounding, your breathing, are the underarms or the palm of your hands sweaty, teeth gritting, fist balling or do you start to physically agitate.

Your lifestyle change will lead you on a path to developing a healthier life. You will be able to balance moment to moment situations as they arise and navigate through life with confidence.

Rose

What about the people, places, things and situations I am confronted with each day?

Therapist

SWEA Tree meditation can be practiced throughout the day.

All you need is your breath and nature.

It is a tension breaker, a rejuvenator, a distraction from negative thoughts, a mind cleanse that releases fear, doubt or any unwanted emotions.

It reduces stress, anxiety and helps with panic attacks.

In time and practice, your subconscious will automatically trigger the breath at the onset of adverse emotions. You will be in a position to receive and let go. That's equivalent to breathing in and breathing out. You will not struggle against the current, rather you will embrace the energy as it flows through.

You do not need to be in a particular setting to meditate or color breathe.

Settings are used for specific matters that you may need to focus on. For instance, you may want to get in the daily habit of meditating. Discover how it feels without distractions around you, create an environment that signals something spiritual is about to take place or simply have a designated space to reinforce daily meditation practice.

With eyes closed to block out distractions, take in deep, slow breaths to the count of three, hold it in for the count of three, and release to the count of three. The counting is mental and serves as a thought distractor. This is a simple and effective approach to releasing stress, anxiety, fear, frustration and panic.

Session #21
(Deep Breathing)

Therapist

Try this:

Sit or stand wherever you are.

Without any pressure, place your hands above your navel.

Breathe naturally.

Make a mental note on how your breathing feels.

Example: Is it fast, short, steady, interrupted?

Keep your hands in place.

Breathe in deeply to a slow mental count of three. Hold your breath to a slow mental count of three. Note the expansion of your diaphragm.

Breathe out slowly to a mental count of three.

While releasing the breath, let your face, mouth, shoulders and upper body relax.

Placing your hands on your diaphragm is mentioned to bring your awareness to how deep you should breathe. You are not stopping your breath midway; you are breathing in deeply enough to cause a slight popped belly. If you feel uncomfortable or dizzy, please discontinue. Take shorter breaths; maybe to the count of two until you are ready to extend your count.

After you get the feel for where your breath will travel, you do not need to continue to keep your hands on your diaphragm.

This should be done throughout the day.

The deep breathing will return you to a state of peace and calm. It will become a habit.

COLOR MEDITATION

COURAGE

Get Up!

Red

Rose

I am afraid that I will die before I start to live. I am afraid I will wake up and my mother would have expired. She has said to me on more than one occasion, "If I don't wake up, I'll be gone." Who says that to their child? I have asked her not to say that, but she eventually says it again. The last time she said it, I told her I love her and to have a good night's sleep. I slept three hours that night and did not go on my usual morning walk. How can I be happy under these circumstances?

Therapist

You are okay to have these fears! Fear will always show itself.

You are feeling helpless because you are not able to predict what your mother will say. When she says things that create fear or anxiety, take a deep breath and release the words with the opposite. "She will wake up in the morning." And smile. Do not allow yourself to hold on to *her* words. They are not your words and they should not be your thoughts. It doesn't matter who dark thoughts come from; they can still create havoc with your emotions. If you are able, dismiss yourself from the room. Sit and take deep breaths. This is an immediate positive reaction to a negative situation.

Your thought of dying before you start to have fun is overpowering the thought of you living and having fun. You have blocked out the visualizations of doing anything for yourself. Your challenge is to create meaningful and fun ways to live. This will require effort on your part. Making a list of low cost and realistic activities should be a priority. Select one activity a week and commit to it the same way you commit to brushing your teeth.

Our fears come from our thoughts. They can be paralyzing, create anxiety, stress, frustration and confusion.

Acknowledging your fear places you in a frame of mind to release it. To let it take its course.

Remember, Yin and Yang. One does not exist without the other. In order to get to the other side, you must be willing to embrace the fear with your breath and release it.

You are afraid because of all the circumstances surrounding you. You are overwhelmed with the stress of caring for your mother, the circumstances in which it occurred, your past trauma and the fact that your life has been turned upside down. Your gauge is on the fear of not being happy or fulfilled. You are stuck there.

In order to move the gauge from unhappy, which is present due to hidden fears about your future, you can approach by using color meditation, deep breathing and visualization. I am including visualization because what you are able to see in your mind as your thoughts are created is powerful and empowering.

Over thinking also causes paralysis. It can keep you confused. Confusion creates mistakes. When mistakes are made, you can become less confident in yourself. Lack of confidence creates your unwillingness to try again. That is fear.

Try not to over think your life. It will keep you guessing.

More often than not, fear will show up. As your life progresses, you will get to feel and recognize how your body responds when you start to feed off fear.

Fear can be helpful, as well. It can alert you and stop you in your tracks. Sometimes stopping will save your life. When we are alerted by our spirit that something is not right and we respond to it in fear, it is usually because we have an unpleasant memory of it happening before.

One of the things you can ask yourself is, "How did I survive it?"

Those memories may come to mind as past trauma or some other occurrence that caused an unhealthy reaction.

Some memories will be recalled as success stories. The success stories are what gives strength to courage. If trauma and other unhealthy emotions outweigh the success stories, fear becomes stronger. The scale tilts in favor of fear.

In any situation with a history of trauma and other fear factors, it is important to create new memories, visualizations, affirmations, actions and stories.

The new visualizations should be based on a desired outcome.

The outcome is held inside of your spirit. It is one of success.

Focus on the goal with your mind, imagination and visualize the outcome.

Remember to not over think what it is you are seeking to accomplish.

Keep your mind and visualization on a successful outcome from beginning to end.

Grounding yourself with courage starts with the understanding of fear and how it relates to you as an individual.

Fear is an emotion that is powerful enough to create paralysis to the mind, body and spirit.

There is a circular motion that connects courage and fear. Just like Yin and Yang, one does not exist without the other. The fear converges into courage and courage converges into fear.

This continuous stream of energy is always present. It is activated with our breath.

The more you meditate and give life to courage, your ability to invoke courage will surface. Fear is still there. You stop feeding it, in other words, stop feeding into it.

You become increasingly aware of your true self and your ability to move the fear out and breathe the courage in. This is a lifetime journey.

Rose

I don't think I have ever thought about breathing and visualization in the way you are discussing it. Can I try a visualization?

Therapist

Yes! Close your eyes. Take slow breaths. Visualize a tree that has been knocked down due to a storm. Do you think the tree is dead or do you think it still has life?

Rose

I don't know how to do that!

Therapist

Try.

Rose

Okay. Give me a minute

It could be dead. Okay, wait! Let me visualize some roots. It won't grow without roots.

Therapist

Continue with your visualization and see it to life. Remember to breathe.

Rose

It is barely alive. I can see a few straggly roots still attached.

Maybe there is hope!

I suppose the roots that are still surviving can get strong again.

Therapist

What will the tree need?

Rose

The tree will need plenty of sun, water, fertile earth and fresh air.

Therapist

Do you think the tree will grow healthy and strong, naturally?

Rose

Yes, I think nature will take its course.

Therapist

Do you think nature will take its course with you?

Rose

Eventually.

Therapist

Open your eyes. I want you to look at this red crystal SWEA tree on the table.

Red evokes courage.

You have more courage than you care to give yourself credit for. Remember how much courage it took to leave an abusive relationship. It took you three or four times to finally rid yourself of the person and situations you feared the most. But, you did it. Once you made up your mind, there was no more straddling the fence.

Each time you are confronted with fear, take a deep breath in, absorbing the energy from the red and imagine that you are grounding yourself with *Courage.*

See your roots planted firmly into the earth.

Breathe out any fear. Breathe in the color red.

Breathe out fear. Breathe in your mission based on a positive visualized outcome.

Continue to focus on the successful task at hand.

Allow the *Red SWEA Tree* to remind you that you are rooted in Courage.

FAITH

───~~~───

Believe!

Orange

I am not certain how this journey will turn out.

I have faith that I will discover ways on how to cope with trauma, depression and anxiety.

I am willing to venture into something that I have never experienced before.

It has to be better than what I have tried in the past.

Self-medicating, eating too much of the wrong foods, sex, unhealthy entertainment and isolation are all failed attempts to deal with my issues. Denying that there is a problem and playing the 'cover up with make-up' game makes me feel horrible and it keeps my vicious cycle of self-abuse going.

What a mess! First someone else abuses me. Then I turn around and do it to myself.

What's the matter with me?

I am desperate to feel better. I am not sure where this therapy with colors and deep breathing will take me, but I must admit, it is different. Also, I like the fact that she is not asking me a million questions about my feelings. Hell, I'm just letting my feelings go without being asked. I feel that she is listening and not judging. Who would have thought talking to a stranger about my life would feel so freeing!

She is sort of letting me tell my story. I also like that she is not sticking to a first, second, and third order of my life line. It doesn't come to me like that.

I am actually starting to believe I will be okay. I am not sure how, but there is something happening inside of me that I am not able to put into words. Maybe because this is new!

So, to you Ms. Therapist, let's have it!

Therapist

Good morning Rose!

Faith is walking through the dark, but believing you are safe and will make it through.

You don't know where you will end up, but it will be the exact place you need to be.

Two choices will be presented. You'll ask yourself, "Should I go this way, or should I go that way?" Regardless to which direction you select, it is important to believe and have faith that it is the correct path. This is not a time to waver and doubt your decision. For example, you knew that the relationship you were in was abusive, so you believed the right thing to do was to leave. You made the decision to leave, but you did not have the faith in yourself to do what you needed to do for yourself and your children. You started to have doubts because you were unable to see your future. You went back to what you were able to see. It didn't matter if it was an abusive relationship or not, it was familiar. It was what you knew.

You began to *straddle the fence.* You fell off the fence when you went back to the relationship. While you were straddling, you were wavering back and forth to doubt and faith or darkness and light. There was something that pushed you over and it was doubt and fear.

Rose, you have walked blindly into so many situations in your life. That final time you left your abuser, you didn't know if he would find you and harm you again. You didn't know how you would feed your children. Somewhere inside of your spirit, you believed that everything was going to be okay. And on top of that, you didn't have a plan. All you wanted to do was to have a safe place for your children and yourself. You crossed over the fence and left doubt and fear behind and believed in something greater than what you were able to see.

Once you start to affirm who you are and what you want to do with your life, meditate and allow your fears and doubts to take its course, your faith will get stronger. You will believe that you will be ok while facing the seemingly impossible.

Something so simple as looking forward to doing something is a lesson in faith. It doesn't matter how big or small it is, it hasn't happened yet. So, how do you know it will happen? A little faith!

You should believe and have faith with the same intensity for the big things as you do for the small things.

There will be times when you will doubt your ability to get through life.

This is normal and also an opportunity to learn about yourself. Ask yourself questions such as, "Why am I doubting?" Don't suppress the answer.

Take some deep breaths, meditate and it will come.

Doubt arrives from lack of self-confidence, listening to other people, or lack of experience in a particular situation. Conclusions start to flood your mind of false endings. You believe in an ending that has been created with fear and it causes you to lack the belief in a positive outcome. Faith is blocked with fear. Faith will evolve once you are able to let the doubt go and breathe in your willingness to let go and let another energy greater than your energy take over.

Sit still and calm yourself with deep breathing for a moment. Take in one slow breath, hold, release and continue that rhythm.

Recall in your mind a time when you successfully completed a task without knowing how it would end.

How did you feel?

Rose

I started thinking about when I made up my mind to not go back to my abuser. Something clicked inside and it was not something I could put my finger on. I was at the lowest point in my life. I didn't know and I wasn't sure of what to do from one moment to the next, but I wasn't afraid, and I believed that my prayers were going to be answered.

I kept moving. I felt stronger and my mind went into a different direction of thought. I began to create ways to make money. Sewing, selling fish sandwiches on Friday nights and babysitting became a way for me to make money.

Therapist

Yes!

Faith is also movement. It does not mean you sit and wait on some miracle to happen. It means doing something to create success.

Close your eyes. I want you to look at that orange SWEA tree on the table. Orange is the spiritual connection to faith.

Each time you are in doubt about something, take in a deep breath. Absorb the energy from the orange and imagine that you are rooted in *faith.* Create an image or story you have survived that was dependent on your ability to remain faithful.

For instance, I am sure that raising your eight children was filled with many challenges. You have a lot to pull from. And what about when your husband went to prison and you were alone and pregnant with five children? How did you do it? It was your faith that got you through the darkness of the unknown.

Breathe in! Imagine your feet planted firmly into the earth. Let the doubt take its course with your out breath. Breathe in and believe that all things are possible. An affirmation of faith would be good to create.

Rose

Okay. *I am not alone.* That's my faith affirmation!

Therapist

I like that!

You may not be able to physically see the end, but you will feel it in your heart. You have affirmed that you are not alone.

Breathe in the color *Orange* and strengthen your spiritual connection with faith.

INTELLECT

─────〜〜〜─────

Messenger

Yellow

Therapist

Right, wrong, not sure why your mind is playing tricks on you?

You can always rationalize why you want to self-medicate or why you don't need to talk to someone. Why you choose to isolate or why you overeat or what's up with all the sweets. It's only sex, I don't want anything serious. But he said he loves me, he promised he'd never do it again. I only get high on the weekend and I always make it up to my children when I'm gone. I need to go on a shopping spree, so what I spent the rent money on a new wardrobe, I deserve it.

The list of justifying irrational decisions are endless.

Our intellect can help or hurt.

Just like everything else, Yin and Yang is present. The universe does not discriminate as it relates to what's right or wrong. We will always arrive at an answer. Whether the answer is favorable or not will depend on what we believe to be true. We can make ourselves believe black is white and white is black. We can justify, rationalize, convince and trick ourselves to believe up is down and down is up.

Our minds are that powerful!

We can see, believe, imagine and create anything within our mundane power. Our minds can be fixed on an idea one moment, and within the next moment it has dissolved. It is our intellect that places us at the crossroads to life. Which way do we go; left or right, up or down, backward or forward or remain where we are? It is the source of all our messages.

When we finally muster up the courage to let go of fear, believing that our situation will get better, we are still faced with a decision as to what to do. Sometimes that *what to do* can disrupt our faith. We believe that things will work in our favor, but sometimes we second guess ourselves. It's our second guessing ourselves that often lead us into hell.

Indecisiveness and irrational actions take over. We become self-imposed victims of fear and doubt. A cycle of mental instability becomes prevalent. We get stuck and go back to our old familiar habits and thoughts.

Akin to our intellect is creativity and inspiration.

Our intellect is how we think and the actions that follow those thoughts. Our thoughts lead to inspiration. Inspiration leads to creation. Visualizations take place of more thoughts and actions. One door opens and another closes. This cycle is endless.

Prayer and affirmations become part of our thought process.

You have heard the saying, "Be careful of what you ask for or pray for."

We will not be able to 'trick' the universe. What we truly believe and ask for will be revealed. When we make a decision, that decision is made based on our thoughts, experiences and emotions. Thoughts change, new experiences emerge, and emotions take their course.

Being mindful of our authentic self and the need to grow in a healthy manner should not be sabotaged with thoughts that are generated with fear, doubt or deceit.

We meditate and deep breathe so that we may also be inspired with new and healthy ideas and to make clear and rational decisions. If a decision doesn't feel right, it isn't right. We should stop convincing ourselves to do something that we know deep down inside our core, isn't right.

Rose, when I am faced with uncertainty, I let it go and give myself 24 hours before I decide. In other words, sleep on it. Once I return to it, I have my answer.

Close your eyes. I want you to look at that yellow SWEA tree on the table. Yellow is the spiritual color that connects to our intellect!

Each time you need to make a decision or if you are in need of inspiration, take a deep breath in and absorb the yellow energy from the yellow SWEA tree.

Use your visualization! Root your feet into the ground and see your hands reaching up and touching yellow rays. Feel the energy as they circulate throughout your entire body.

Affirm your willingness and ability to make rational decisions.

Allow your thoughts and visualizations to redirect and place you back on course with clarity.

Breathe out indecisiveness, breathe in and focus on your decision.

See and believe what you are affirming.

Breathe in the *Yellow and be inspired!*

BALANCE

Mind, Body, Spirit!

Green

Therapist

Our willingness and ability to clear our negative energy and replace it with healthy thoughts, prayers and affirmations, create a strong body by eating healthy foods and engage in physical activities, and to calm our spirit with our in and out breath, is a lifelong journey.

Green is the color that is used for meditation to accomplish this goal.

With the balance and unconditional love green expresses, we become less stressed, depressed and depleted. As we breathe in the energy from this color, our spirit connection starts to work in harmony with our mind, body and spirit.

We naturally gravitate to ways and means that are beneficial for our *Whole Self.*

For example, that walk in the park is no longer a simple walk. Your spirit has started the process of balancing the Whole Self with each breath that is taken while walking through the park. Sort of like being in an intensive care environment for balance. Food choices will start to include more green foods and your energy level will improve. Your acknowledgment of unconditional love for self will resonate with your spirit. You will become aware of a deeper love for self rather than on the surface. That love for self helps with relaxation, rejuvenation and restorative energies.

Our breath is our healthy life. Green balances our mind, body and spirit.

Let's look at the role of the other colors we have meditated with for a moment.

Red, orange and yellow can be referred to as colors with objective energy. In other words, they are the colors that get us moving. Red gets us going, orange keeps us moving and yellow inspires. We need all three colors to work in harmony.

From a different perspective, red also represents our body, orange represents our spirit and yellow our mind. They must also work in harmony.

It is the color green that we need to keep our *Whole Self* (mind, body, spirit) balanced.

For example: Too much exercise and not enough mental stimulation can create an imbalance. The goal is to balance taking care of our body, mind and spirit as close as we can with equal attention. Eat healthy and exercise, think positive and affirm who you are and breathe.

This is the purpose for meditating with the green SWEA tree.

Green is unconditional. What we do and think is who and what we become.

When we are balanced everything changes.

We start to get better, feel better and do better for ourselves and others.

Colors do not discriminate. They are global. Red is red in Australia and the Caribbean.

Unconditional love is the ultimate aspect of green and it does not discriminate.

When we achieve balance, our lifestyle, thoughts, actions, what we do for others and how we treat ourselves, changes. Our overall health changes.

Green is balanced unconditional love and growth.

Meditate with the *Green SWEA Tree* for balance and unconditional love of self. Bring balance into your mind, body and spirit.

EXPRESSION

Communicate

Aqua

Therapist

We are who you are.

Our language, culture, dance, facial expressions, gestures, our touch, silence, likes, dislikes, occupations, how we socialize, and who we socialize with are a few examples of how we present ourselves to the world.

How we communicate ourselves to the world is a sum total of our life experiences, our family environment and is constantly changing with each thought.

Expression involves our total communication of mind, body and spirit. We are not able to hide who we are, even when we try.

You've heard the saying, *"The truth of who we are will always come to the light."*

Change is constantly in motion. It is created inward and flows outward. During the journey back into our spirit, we sometimes bring back other folk's expressions or communications of what they think of us, who they think we should be, how they think we should act and a host of other adverse messages that create a false sense of who we are.

We are sometimes referred to as being 'fake'. Also, we don't know who we are and become confused and our self-esteem suffers.

We sometimes transform ourselves into what we think folks wants us to be, in an effort to please them and to be liked.

Without the balance of courage, faith and a clear head, we tend to lose confidence.

We need balance in order to help with the true expression of who we are.

Once balance is achieved, we naturally evolve to a higher level of consciousness.

The aqua SWEA Tree is the color where we ground ourselves with a clear communication of our divine purpose and the manner in which we communicate and express our authentic self.

In comparison to yellow, which is also a communication color, aqua is steadfast, whereas yellow wavers. They both are vital. One is not better than the other. They represent the Yin and Yang of the energy centers as it relates to communication.

The Divinity of our true expression is manifested when we meditate using the breathing and visualization of *aqua*. We breathe in the calming color of aqua to achieve this goal.

Meditate with the *Aqua SWEA Tree* in order to discover your divine purpose, the manner in which you express your purpose and your willingness to communicate.

AWARENESS

Insight

Indigo

Therapist

Secret resentments of anger and resentments aimed at people who are unable to hear you, will destroy you.

With Indigo, we become aware of our so-called hidden secrets that we think have disappeared.

In the midnight hour, we are sometimes awakened by a dream that reveals to us a truth that we may or may not be ready for. It is truthfully revealing, but not at that exact moment.

Our awareness is an intuitive energy that is subtle and affirmative. We get shifted into a rim of thoughtlessness and rely on what is being transmitted from a source that exceeds our comprehension. If we try to force ourselves to use logic, we lose the essence of the energy. When we doubt, we block the natural energy of our insight to the unknown.

Awareness is kin to faith. We have faith without seeing, but we can let doubt muddy our faith. Awareness is the divine level of insight that is not questioned or attached to any emotion.

As we evolve into our authentic selves through prayer, deep breathing, meditation and our affirmations, our insight about who we are, situations and the world, changes.

We are able to know without being told or having answers before us. We rely on our insight and intuitively see things which may or may not be in front of our eyes.

Awareness is more than knowledge or intellect.

Awareness cannot be taught from books. It happens randomly, but through meditation it can be recognized and strengthened on the spiritual level. Our breath helps us to use our insight at will.

As we evolve, the energy from this color is manifested in our ability to rely on our insight when it is needed. Meditate with the *Indigo SWEA Tree.*

Wisdom

Truth

Purple

Therapist

Our truth, is our journey and our journey, is our truth.

The color purple represents our entire life as an evolved self-living and sharing life based on truth.

Our path is embedded within our spirit.

Our choices are determined by the total of our life's experiences.

Wise decisions are based on our ability to live truthfully, free of emotion or influence.

Wisdom is truth. Emotions are taken out of the equation when faced with decisions.

Emotions such as fear, doubt and indecisiveness block wisdom.

Truth does not lie. If you have lived a life inflicting harm to others, that is part of your journey.

If you have lived a life helping others, that is part of your journey.

When truth is altered, it is not truth. Wisdom evolves from your true life. Anything other than that will be a lie. A lie unfolds because of an emotion.

Wisdom is void of emotions and *is what it is!*

As we age, we strive to learn from our mistakes. Sometimes, we repeat the same lessons over and over again. When we finally *get it,* our entire mindset changes on that particular matter. We have entered the age of wisdom.

Living a life based on Yin is truth and living a life based on Yang is also truth.

Telling your story correctly and making decisions without emotions is wisdom. It does not matter what the subject is. Wisdom is real stories from true life experiences.

It does not discriminate or indicate or distinguish good from bad.

Right or wrong, folks make what is considered wise decisions based on their individual journey.

Wisdom is absent of fear, logic and doubt.

Meditating with the color purple develops the ability to use wisdom. It will help you arrive at a wise decision absent of emotions. Life experiences evolve into wisdom. If you do not have life experiences, seek an elder or spiritual advisor.

The color purple has the healing and spiritual energy of helping make wise decisions based on truth rather than emotions.

Meditate with the *Purple SWEA Tree.*

PEACE

Omnipresent

Transparent

Therapist

Our ability to breathe in peace and breathe out every thought and emotion.

Unconditional love of everything, all the time.

Peace in the presence of adversity.

Meditate with transparent when you want to let go of mental clutter, confusion and every emotional disruption you can possibly think of. It is the equivalent to a spiritual laxative. It releases so that the ability to start again is possible. It is our breath.

Meditate with transparent when you need to release all the noise in your head that you are not sure where it's coming from. Meditate with this transparent SWEA Tree to simply, let go.

The Yin and Yang of color

Yin – Yang

Red – Purple

Orange – Indigo

Yellow – Aqua

Green balances the Yin and the Yang

THE SWEA TREE

SWEA Tree Meditation (Sun, Water Earth and Air)

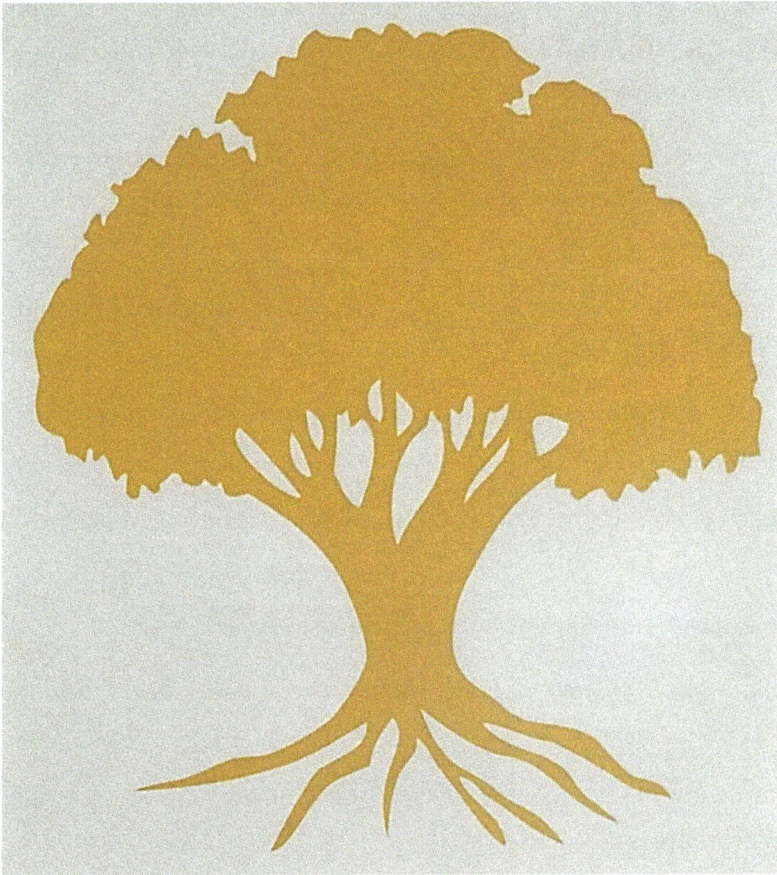

The seven roots connected to the SWEA Tree represents the seven energy centers.

These centers are also referred to as Chakras, which is a Sanskrit term that translates to energy centers.

The SWEA Tree is yellow. Yellow represents inspiration and intelligence. It also represents the Sun.

We are never without the energy centers.

We have a major and minor energy that is our spiritual *go to* color energy.

It can be thought of as your favorite and second favorite color. If you don't have a favorite color, that's quite alright! It will reveal itself through meditation.

Everyone's essence makes up the same colors, but in varying degrees. For instance, I may manifest blue as my dominant expression, whereas you may manifest red. This is how color works in its simplest form.

The unifying fact is, without any thought, we breathe in and out energy created from the sun, water, earth and air.

Our life goal is to prevent, maintain and heal ourselves using natural remedies.

Energy from the sun, water, earth and air will alleviate diseases of the mind, body and spirit.

We strive to work in harmony with nature.

Basic necessities such as food, shelter, herbs, water and clothing are obtained from earth.

Clean and unpolluted air and water, the sun and earth are essential for our existence.

SWEA Tree Meditation *Wholistic (Wholistic embodies the whole person, the entire planet and natural solutions to healing the mind, body and spirit)* provides a natural path using color and nature to foster a healthy mind, body and spirit.

When we care for our *Whole* self, we begin to gravitate towards a better method of caring for self. We start to make health-conscious decisions deriving from nature.

Eating a diet composed of healthy foods from the earth is essential for optimal health and wellness.

When we deviate from natural foods, our body, mind and spirit are being deprived of creating a healthy relationship with earth.

When we take in healthy foods with our diet, exercise or have healthy thoughts, we evolve into healthy individuals. This is the gateway to expressing our authentic selves, becoming aware of our life's purpose and to live our lives based on truth and wisdom.

This is not to say we must be a vegetarian or never eat potato chips, ice cream or cake.

However, if you have an unhealthy addiction to foods that have been processed or slathered with sugar, salt or other unhealthy additives, it is wise to create limits and find healthier choices.

Salt, sugar, fats, and carbohydrates are highly addictive; search for alternatives.

Moving your body is vital. Our bodies are meant to move to avoid dis-eases. Movement creates strong muscles, helps with the circulation and regulation of the fluids in our body, helps with our breathing, and is good for our lungs and heart; the bottom line is that movement is a *whole* experience for the entire body, mind and spirit.

You do not need to become an exercise fanatic, but you do need to become aware of your lack of movement and what it does to your body.

Get started with a walk. Walking is underestimated.

Deep breathing and color meditation are natural remedies that aid in healing our mind, body and spirit. When we breathe in and meditate with the color orange for example, we are transmitting to our spirit that we are in need of faith, which is the absence of doubt. You may say, "I'm good, everything is going okay in my life." At that moment, it may be true, however the amazing thing about our essence is that we may not consciously know about a situation that is coming, but somehow the soul of who we are knows and prepares us for it, just as we prepare for the possibility of a storm. That orange, or faith that we meditate with is like money in our spiritual bank.

We will be able to use the energy at will because we have prepared ourselves.

This is how your major and minor colors can be looked at. They are the colors that will keep surfacing, if you allow them to.

It takes practice to develop insight and use them in time of need.

This is how the SWEA Tree is used for deep breathing and meditation.

For those who are not sure which color to start with, start with the transparent SWEA Tree.

This is equivalent to clearing the slate. You are letting go of any un-wanted energy that clutter, confuse or harbor negative emotions.

It is the gateway to peace and love.

The Tree of *Peace* SWEA Tree is great for anyone starting meditation or deep breathing for the first time.

Being consistent is important for success. Deep breathing and medita-tion should be approached as a part of your daily routine.

Why a SWEA Tree Symbol?

Symbols have always aided in helping with memory. Trees are rooted in the earth and reminds us to keep ourselves grounded. We need the same water, earth, air and sun as the tree. Trees provide oxygen and represent longevity, growth and resurrection.

The seven roots are a reminder that we are rooted in the earth with the seven energy centers.

Red, orange and yellow are energies from the sun. Aqua, indigo and purple from the ocean.

Emerald and forest green plant life from the earth. The transparency of air.

Plant life and flowers surround us with vibrant colors. There is nature all around us. Flowering trees, fruit trees, trees, seashells, rocks, driftwood, lakes, ponds, snow, rain, mountains, vines, rivers and waterfalls, stars, clouds, grass, sand, ocean, moon, stars, flowers, leaves.

THE SEVEN SWEA TREES

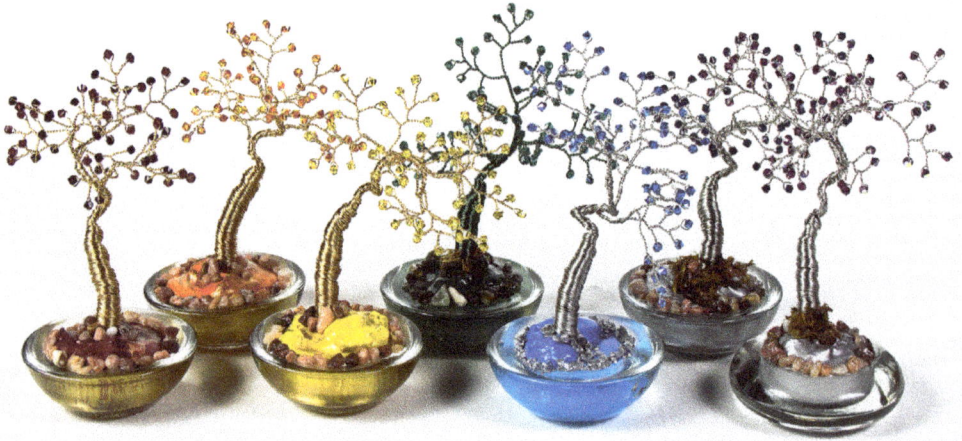

Courage, Faith, Intellect, Balance, Expression,
Awareness and Wisdom.

Red - Courage

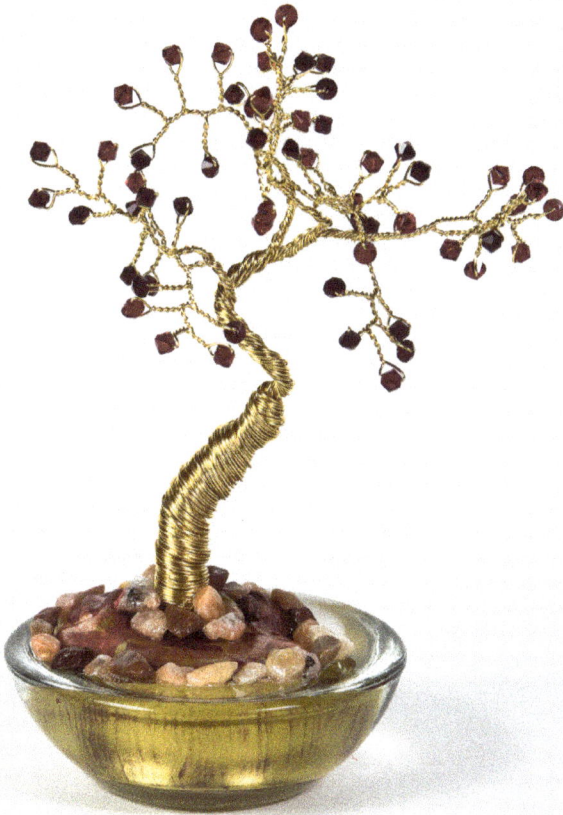

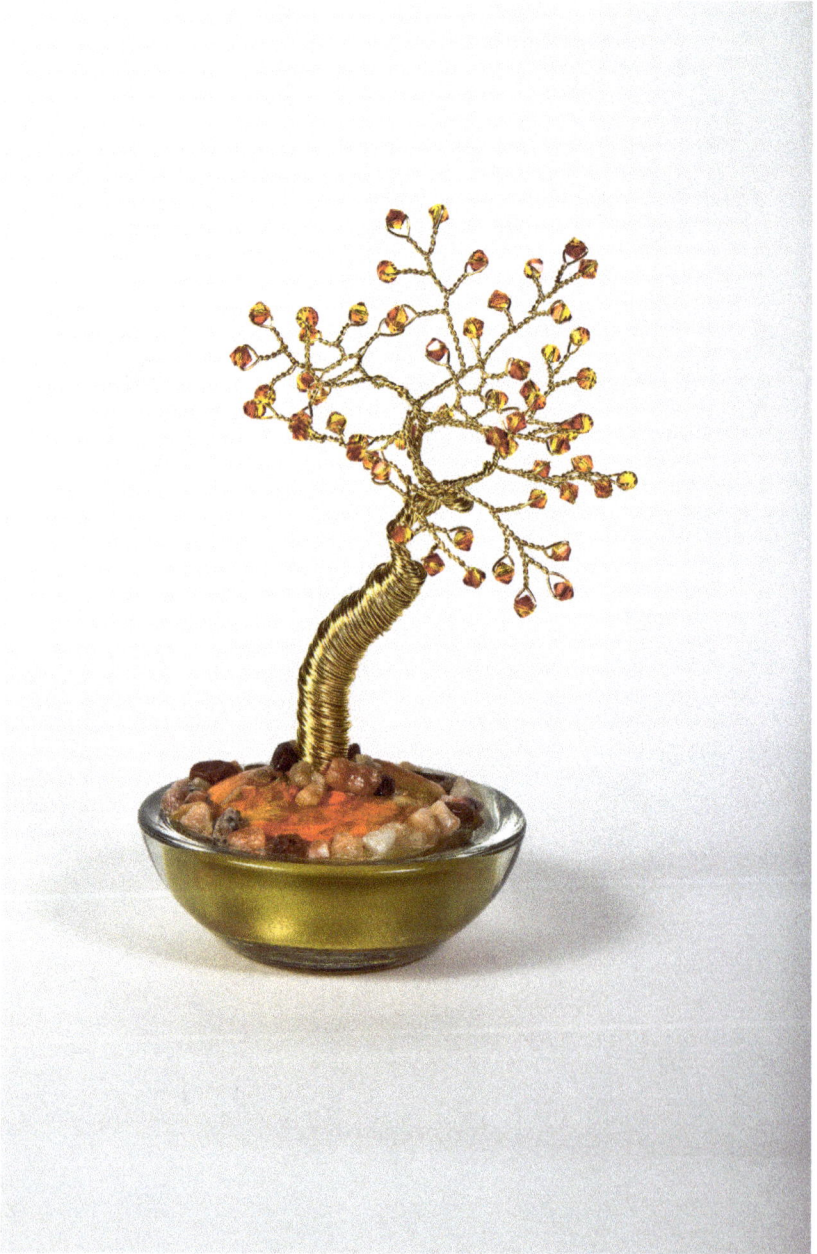

Orange - Faith

Yellow - Intellect

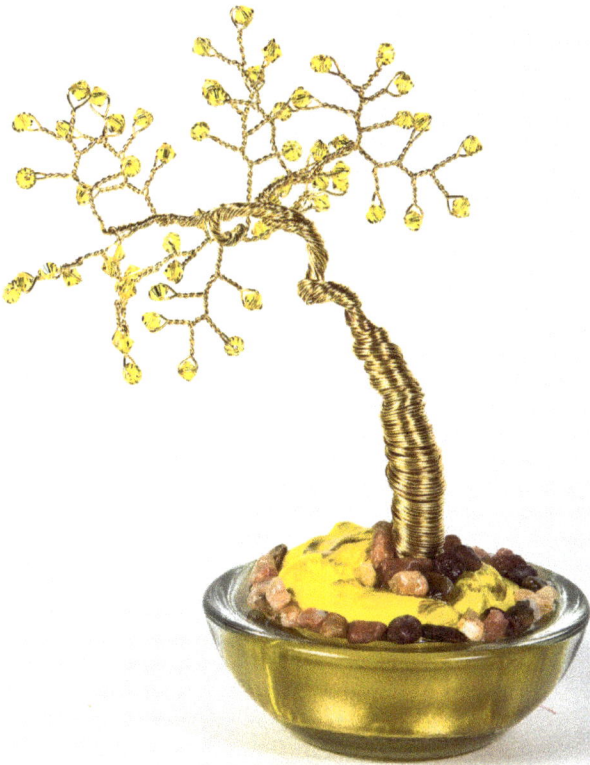

Green - Balance

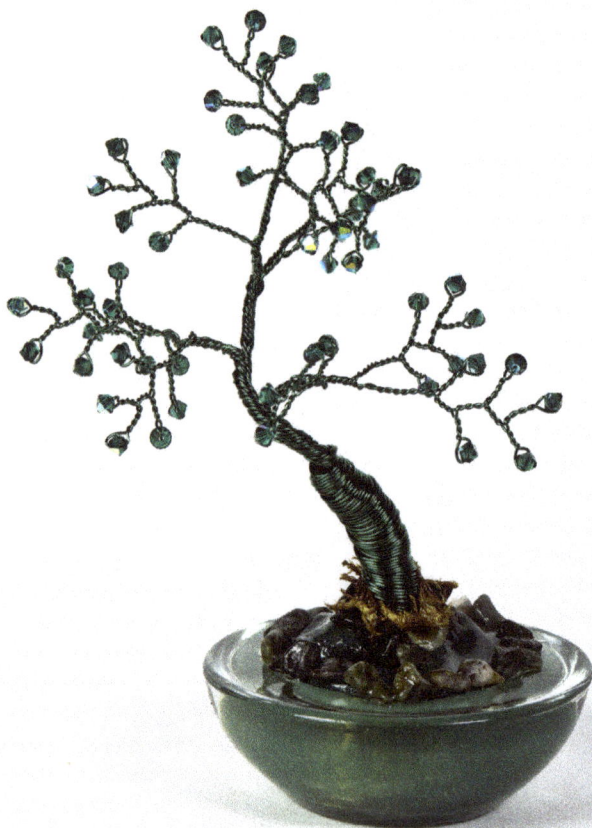

Aqua - Expression

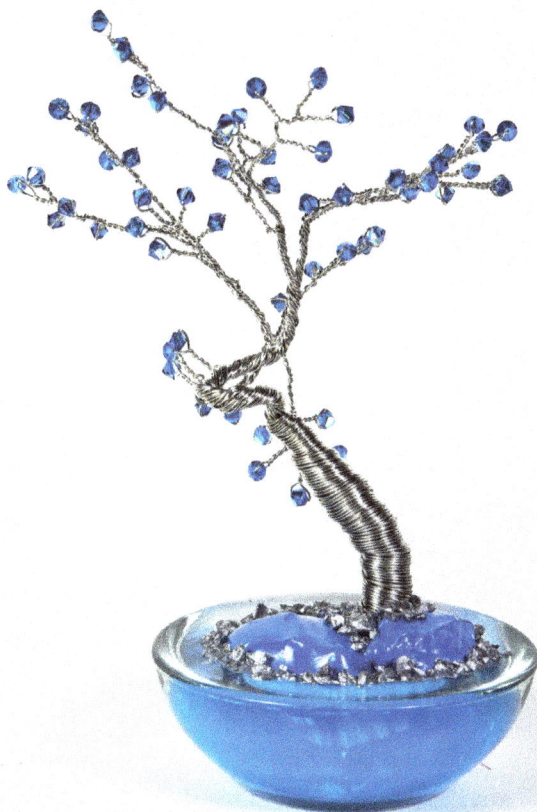

Indigo - Awareness

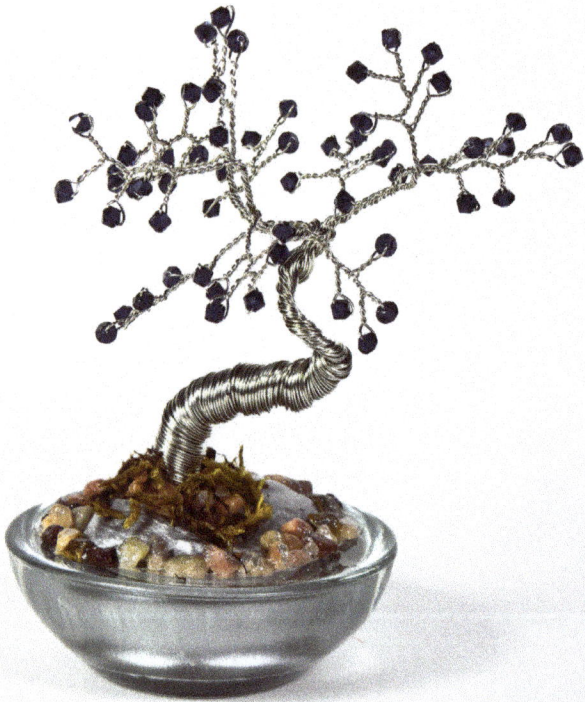

Purple - Wisdom

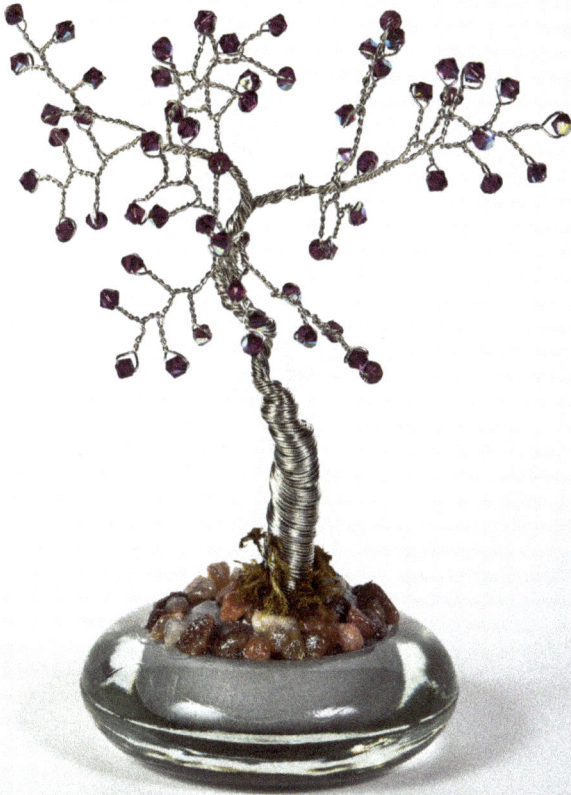

White - Peace

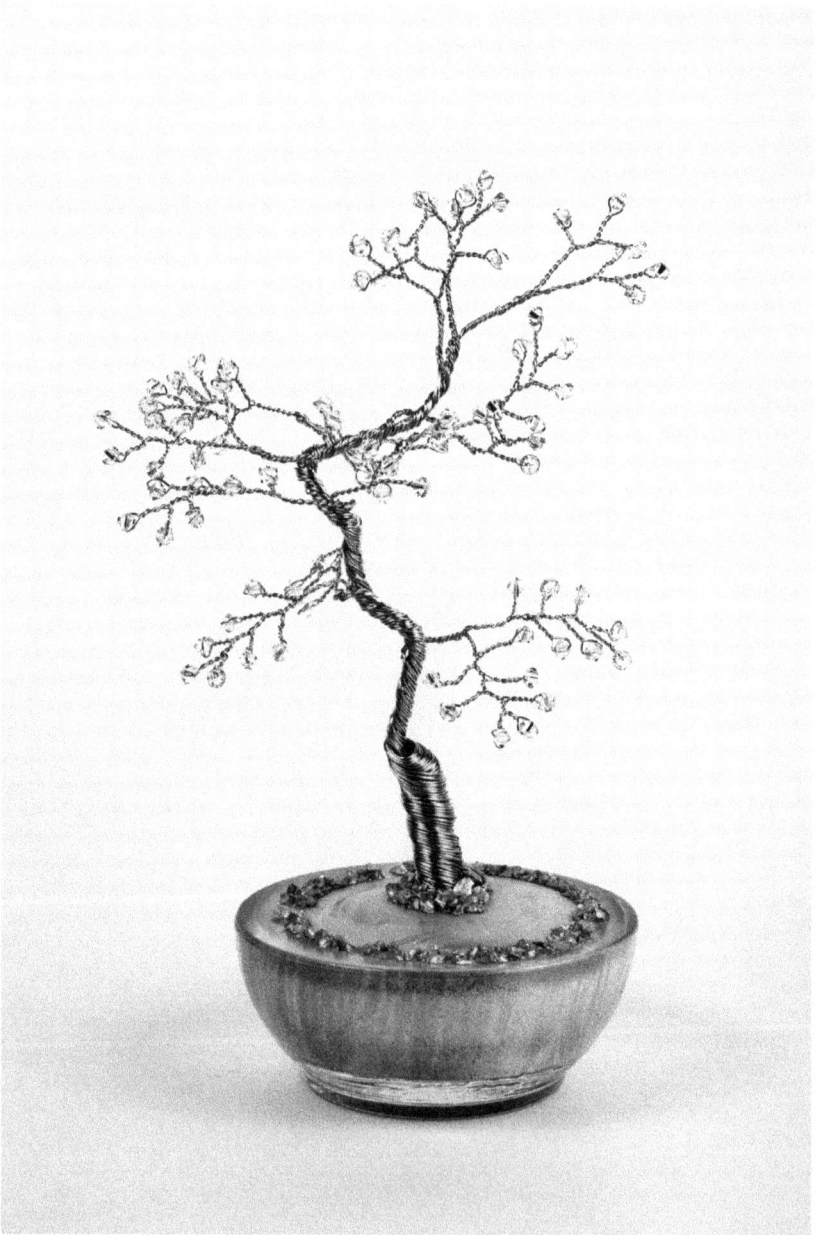

SOMEWHERE IN A RAINBOW

Gems

Every prayer that you pray has already been answered.

I am my Affirmation.

Colors lie within.

Take a Break.

Go for a walk.

Listen to someone today.

Forgive someone today.

Relax your mind and your body, breathe.
Forgive yourself today.

"They only come around when they need something."
Thank heaven they come around. Be the light that you are.

Having someone to go to for help is a blessing for the giver and the receiver.
Having someone come to you for help is a blessing for the receiver and the giver.

Our purpose of forgiveness is to heal our body, mind and spirit.

Breathe deeply.

Courage has no fear.

Meditate with a healing purpose in mind.

Breathe in and get it.

Your feelings are what wake you up in the morning and put you to sleep at night.
They are a part of your everything!
They say, "Don't feel that way!"
You say, "But I do feel this way."
Allowing yourself to process your feelings will expose it for what it is; a moment in your life of living. Our thoughts are like a river, constantly flowing.
Feel more and breathe more.
Avoid a buildup. Breathe it out and allow yourself to let it go!

Our feelings are an indicator that we are alive.

We are connected to a Higher Source of love and light.
Light keeps us out of the dark. Our belief in a Higher Source grounds our faith in knowing and feeling that there is an omnipresent and infinite amount of love and light.

Things and possessions are not the Ultimate Source for Happiness.

Dream, Believe, Plan & Do It!

Breathe in nature.

Breathe in color.

Thinking about and imagining ourselves in someone else's life situation is an awareness that teaches us how to be compassionate and understanding. It inspires and motivates us to reach out and help in ways that we are able to help, rather than stand back, point fingers and criticize.

Uncover a fun and rejuvenating experience!

We need mental & spiritual grounding throughout our day. Stop and take deep breaths.
Let go of all the unhealthy clutter, chatter, visuals, toxic thoughts and memories.
Place deep breathing on your "to do" list. Stop and breathe in and out, seven deep breaths at various times throughout the day.

Change starts with courage and the willingness to change.

When a family member goes to a prison facility for punishment, it affects the family.

Preventing, managing and maintaining a healthy mind, body and spirit takes a lifetime.

Find 365 reasons and ways to LOVE yourself.

Think it, Create it, Do it.

Find something fun and meaningful to do.

Make a list of things to look forward to doing.

Laugh and smile more.

Let go of those hurtful, angry, resentful and selfish thoughts.
Replace them each with loving, kind and caring thoughts.

Don't straddle the fence.

Ask for Help.

A spiritual laxative is just as important as a physical.

Something that is growing inside is taking on a life of its own. It has been growing all the time.

Use your natural gifts to lift yourself up. It will also lift others.

Meditation and deep breathing strengthen your spiritual immune system.

Wholesome and healthy foods strengthen your physical immune system.

Positive thoughts and affirmations strengthen your mental immune system.

When inconsiderate words filled with pain and hurt come from someone, don't retaliate with the same energy. Rather, give yourself healthy thoughts and if possible, remove yourself from the situation.

Get Help.

Courage has no fear.

Sip some tea.

Feel Better.

While walking remember to breathe.

I am doing better! I am feeling better! I am getting better!

Don't hold all those "hating on someone" stories in your head. They will become your reality and create stress and dis-ease.

There will be times when sitting or lying down is all you are able to do.
Your energy is depleted.
You may feel a silent gentle force lifting you up!
You walk to the bathroom, turn the shower to warm and step under the running water.
The sound of the water and the feeling on your body revives you
Someone dresses you.
Your hand is held, and you are guided out the door.
Maybe you walk through the neighborhood, sit on a beach or walk through a park.
You may even talk to God.

Don't allow someone to share their toxic energy with you. Dismiss yourself and them.

Holding on to negative thoughts is like holding on to physical waste in our bodies.
Eventually we will need a laxative to get rid of the waste.
Meditation and deep breathing are our spiritual laxative.
Senna is a good laxative for the body.

Get some rest.

Make caring for your health and well-being a PRIORITY!

Create a list.
Do not put an unrealistic number of things to do on it.
Putting too many things to do on a list can overwhelm you if you're not able to complete the list.

Don't get overwhelmed with the thought of being overwhelmed!
Thinking about all the things that must be done is
OVERWHELMING!!!

Prioritize one goal at a time! Whether it is finances, chores, work or a health issue. The number one thing to remember is that you are able to only do one thing at a time. Our mind is strong and can sometimes play tricks on us to believe that we can do a number of things at once. We eventually become stressed and run ourselves into a wall of frustration.

Don't flood your mind with so much to do. The thought of so many things to do is exhausting and perpetuates feelings of being overwhelmed and anxious and creates anxiety and stress.

Create a once a week habit of avoiding: Emails, Social Media, News Reports, Unnecessary Texting & Phone calls. Your family and friends will be fine if you step away for a day. Better a day than a week or months recovering from a major illness that could have been prevented with a little of self-care.

Awareness and devotion to our purpose will promote a healthy mind, body and spirit.

Say NO! You do not need to always say YES! No explanation necessary.

Select one day each week to eliminate distractions. Use this day to meditate with a transparent or white SWEA Tree. Breathe in the aroma of Lavender or Lotus oil to enhance deep breathing.

Allow yourself to PRIORITIZE yourself each day of your life, in some way!

Make healthy foods a PRIORITY!

Make your life a PRIORITY!

Unhealthy and traumatic life situations create mentally and spiritually unstable individuals if proper healing remedies are not put in place. When the mind and spirit suffer, the body also becomes unstable. Unstable individuals that we come into contact with often end up hurting us verbally, physically and even with the silent treatment. It is not always the intention of a person to hurt someone else, but there is truth in the words, "Hurt people."

It is traumatic when a child is bullied, witnesses domestic violence, abandoned, neglected emotionally, verbally abused, physically assaulted or sexually violated.

Once this happens, it cannot unhappen. The child lives this trauma everyday of their life. It can lie dormant and be triggered by certain situations, people, places, smells, things and a host of occurrences that sparks an unhealthy behavior in response to the trauma.

As their age progresses, outlets such as substance abuse, sexual promiscuity, violence, self-abuse, workaholism, alcoholism, and isolation become coping behaviors.

Deep within, the individual feels unhappy and knows that something isn't right.

The thought never occurs, "Maybe I should seek professional help."

Seeking professional help would be a clear indicator that something is the matter and who would want to admit that!

More than likely, there is a friend who co-signs the behaviors or ignores it. Afterall, friends do not want to hurt the feelings of a friend.

Each day, life is continuing to load unresolved problems, issues and situations.

Low self-worth, lack of faith, irrational decisions and fear are symptoms that are generated.

Stress becomes a way of living and depression often settles in.

Upset feelings and anger over small things comes easily.

Fatigue, insomnia, irritability, and frustration also become constants.

The day to day living episodes create other problems such as headaches, digestion problems, hypertension and muscle tension.

On occasion, they take a yoga or meditation class, go on vacation, have a night out with friends, spiritual retreats, NA, AA or religious services.

However, there is still this knot in their throat. They know they are doing things and speaking, but they feel as though they are not being heard or understood.

The decades of saying, "I'm good" when someone asks how they feel is no longer working. They realize that they are not "good." They are living a lie!

On the outside, they seem okay to friends, family and peers.

On the inside, they are crying and hurting.

Alternative or traditional therapy is vital in order to help unravel the core cause to mental and spiritual distress.

21 Affirmations

21 days of affirmations create healthy habits. Start creating!

1.

2.

3.

4.

5.

6.

7.

8.

9.

10.

11.

12.

13.

14.

15.

16.

17.

18.

19.

20.

21.

About the Author

There is no limit to the amount of descriptives 1 could use that would totally describe Rasheedah Sharif aka Ma-me. Beautiful-Serious-Intelligent-Strong- Fearless-Creative-Driven and a Survivor are just a few words that come to mind.

My mother single handedly raised eight biological children and many others with barely any assistance from anyone, yet never questioned God nor complained. I learned from my mother that a person's limitations are only stifled by their inability to imagine. In a world that can be full of discourse and chaos, my mother taught us (her children) how to unearth a sacred space within our self to find peace and balance. Rasheedah Sharif is truly my "She-Ro", mentor, friend, but most importantly, my Ma-me.

Shakira

R….REAL

A….Artist

S….Smart

H….Honest

E….Energetic

E….Earthly

D….Delicate

A….Amazing

H….Healthy

S….Serious

H….Happy

A….African-American

R….Rich

I….Intelligent

F….Fun

Less is MORE, so I used ONE word for each letter of my mommy's name to share the characteristics of Rasheedah Sharif, my mother, mentor, friend, and inspiration! Thank you, Mommy for showing us how to make a goal and ACHIEVE IT!!!

Maryam

As long as I can remember, my mother, "Sister Rasheedah" was always determined and consistent in serving the youth and raising her children. Educating the youth was her Divine Mission. She is also a wonderful writer and actress. She played a role in a play, *For Colored Girls who have Considered Suicide When the Rainbow is Enuf.* She was the color brown. She had an opportunity to continue her acting but she chose to put her time, money and passion into the youth.

She started writing and directing her own plays and let the youth act them out. She also had an opportunity to run for council woman. She chose not to because her passion was with the youth.

Now, she wrote her second book. I pray and I know that she will have great success.

She's one of God's great, best kept secrets.

Love always, your son, Messiah.

What can I say about Rasheedah Sharif as an author? She's amazing!!! Her book *Don't Come Down from the Chinaberry Tree* was truly motivational for me. Regardless of what the character Rose went through, she made it and her story helped me get through my own personal journey. One of the quotes that I absolutely love is "been through the mill but didn't get grinned up." Rasheedah's stories and blogs keep me motivated, her words give me the courage to walk through life with my head held high and my feet firmly on the ground. Rasheedah Sharif is an extraordinary AUTHOR/ WOMAN/ MOTIVATIONALIST/ MOTHER/ ARTIST, she is and always will be my SHERO!!

Yaya

It's really a blessing to be able to see my mother follow her dreams. Be creative with her entrepreneurial skills. It was fashion, fashion shows, all different types of art, a book, teaching. It was always something productive. As a young boy, I didn't understand how resilient and determined you were, but now it's clear. You were and still are a true Warrior. As a mother of 8, you made it look easy from my perspective. I'm also the #7 child, so by that time you might have mastered motherhood. All that to say I witnessed greatness!

Imani

As I am sitting here, thinking about all the wonderful things I can say about my mother, my mind is drawing a blank. Not because I have nothing to say, but because there is nothing I can say that will truly encompass the magnitude of her greatness. During my twenty-seven years of life, she has been my mother, my teacher, my confidant, my role model, my friend, and my hero. I have watched my Ma'Me selflessly extend her wisdom and heart towards her community through teaching, counseling, mentoring, and creating beautiful safe spaces to allow creativity and talent to grow. She is everything I aspire to be. Words cannot express how much I am proud of her and how thankful I am that the Universe has chosen me to be her daughter.

Thank you, Ma'Me. I love you so much. You are phenomenal.

Your Chi

Therapist

What would you do if you were high in the mountains, in a tiny room with no windows or doors?

Rose

I think I'd just find me a spot to sit, close my eyes, breathe and stay alive.

Rasheedah Sharif, Wholistic Artist

Master Level Therapist

Certified Domestic Violence Advocate

SWEA Tree Color Meditation

Deep Breathing Meditation

SWEA Tree Art for Meditation

Narrative Therapy

CONTACT

www.rasheedahsharif.com

Instagram@growingsweatrees

Facebook/Rasheedahsharif.com

YouTube/Rasheedah Sharif

rasheedah@sweatree.com